What the healing community is saying....

"Laura Davis has written a gentle, compassionate and affirming book. *Allies in Healing* is a gift to the millions who struggle as partners of survivors."

> — Stephanie S. Covington, Ph.D.
> coauthor of *Leaving the Enchanted Forest* and
> author of *Awakening Your Sexuality*

"The significance of this book as a tool for communication between partners cannot be overstated. *Allies in Healing* offers a guide to previously uncharted territories for both partners to resolve together."

> —Hank Estrada
> PLEA
> Santa Fe, New Mexico

"Once again Laura Davis has come up with a timely and supportive book about healing from sexual abuse. Partners can now feel supported and guided in their quest for healing—for themselves and for those they love and cherish."

> —Dan Sexton
> Childhelp USA
> National Survivors of Child Abuse Program

"Among the healthy proliferation of new books in the field of sexual abuse, *Allies in Healing* is one of the most urgently needed. I am relieved to finally have an intelligent, sensitive, and supportive book to recommend to partners who are struggling to take care of themselves and to help the survivors they love. Partners deserve help, too. *Allies in Healing* gives help that is honest, practical, and true."

> —Ellen Bass
> coauthor of *The Courage to Heal* and
> coeditor of *I Never Told Anyone*

"Even if *Allies in Healing* wasn't provocative, compelling, deeply sensitive, and—at moments—funny, it would still be a valuable addition to the literature of healing. But it is all of these things. Laura Davis has done it again."

> —Geneen Roth
> author of *When Food is Love, Breaking Free,*
> and *Feeding the Hungry Heart*

"Laura demonstrates a level of professionalism and understanding of sexual molestation issues that far exceeds anything I have read or been taught."

—Camille Caiozzo, Ph.D.
clinical psychologist
Los Angeles, California

What partners and survivors are saying. . . .

"I carry *Allies in Healing* around with me everywhere. My boyfriend had to go out and buy his own copy. I couldn't bear to part with mine."

—partner from Colorado

"My wife and I consider your book our second Bible."

—partner from Texas

"Your books have saved my marriage and my life. From the bottom of my heart, thank you."

—survivor from Louisiana

"I have had your book for five hours. I have read it for twenty minutes. I have broken down sobbing twice. I am now taking a break to thank you."

—partner from California

"It was wonderful to see you talk. You were eloquent, funny, honest and again and again, courageous. I am delighted by the way you champion a voice for survivors and partners. You are an inspiration."

—survivor from Massachusetts

"I've been in treatment since I was six. I've been in mental hospitals. I've been given shock treatments. I've been on meds. I've seen counselors up the wazoo, but this was the first real help I've ever received."

—survivor from New Jersey

"Your presence is strong, compassionate, reassuring. I received hope and strength—a vision for myself."

—partner from New York

"Thank you! Thank you! Thank you! Finally we know we are not alone."

—two-survivor couple from Oregon

ALLIES IN
HEALING

WHEN THE PERSON YOU LOVE WAS
SEXUALLY ABUSED AS A CHILD

LAURA DAVIS

wm

WILLIAM MORROW

An Imprint of HarperCollins Publishers

In memory of Scott Chase
July 1954 - October 1991
whose contribution to this
book made a difference.

Designed by Laura Hough

Library of Congress Cataloging-in-Publication Data

Davis, Laura.
   Allies in healing: when the person you love was sexually abused as a child / Laura Davis.—1st HarperPerennial ed.
      p.   cm.
   Includes bibliographical references and index.
   ISBN 0-06-055299-9 (cloth) — ISBN 0-06-096883-4 (paper)
   1. Adult child sexual abuse victims—Mental health.
2. Interpersonal relations.   I. Title.
RC569.5.A28D38   1991
616.85′83—dc20   90-56423

---

50 49 48 47 46   (pbk)

To my Partner,
Karyn Bristol

CONTENTS

PART II: **PARTNERS' STORIES**

ACKNOWLEDGMENTS

For the last several years, I have had the opportunity and privilege to lead workshops for partners of survivors around the country. I am extremely grateful to the men and women who came to these workshops and shared their stories, frustrations, courage, and pain. Their hunger for information and their willingness to share formed the basis of this book. Thanks, too, to the authors of the questions which make up so much of this book.

I'd also like to thank:

My readers, Ellen Bass, Susan Bryer, Abe Davis, Susan Frankel, Paula Inwood, Cecily Knepprath, Jim Malone, Leilani Miller, Celine Marie Pascal, Amy Pine, Keith Rand, Geneen Roth, Shauna Smith, and Stephanie Smith, for excellent suggestions and feedback.

My editor, Janet Goldstein, for clear thinking and inspiration.

Her assistant, Peternelle van Arsdale, for encouragement and support.

My literary agent, Charlotte Raymond, and lecture agents, Denise Notzon and Jaimee Karroll, for humor, good conversation, and help getting this work into the world.

The producers of The Courage to Heal workshops, whose hard work and vision gave me the chance to develop and refine this material. Along with the volunteers who put in countless hours, I'd like to thank: Dino Sierp, Nona Gandelman and Lynn Goulder, Libby Harman and Joan Levin, Susan Stiles Wilson and the folks at Greenbriar Hospital, Darcey Spears, Dorothy Peterson, Maxine Stein and the folks at the Women's Resource Center, Barbara Debes, Sally

Palain, Tam Martin, Denise Wheeler, Cecily Knepprath, Charlotte Watson, Sue Estler and the University of Maine, Linda Shirley, Jean Vogel, Louise Bauschard and the St. Louis Women's Self-Help Center, Carol Meade and Iowa CASA, Gayle Stringer and King County Rape Relief, Catherine Ratte and Wisconsin CASA, Harriet Pickett, Havens Levitt and Wimin in Movement in New Mexico.

The following partners and survivors: Tom and Fran Okerlund, Angela Gleason, Shelly Skye, Scott Chase, and Jim Fereira.

My professional colleagues for encouragement, clarity, and belief in this project: Lynn Bryant, Mimi Farrelly, Randy Fitzgerald, Hank Estrada, Susan Frankel, Eliana Gil, Paul Hansen, Thom Harrigan, Richard Jacobs, Paul Kimmel, Laurel King, Mike Lew, Wendy Maltz, Robin Moulds, Carol Plummer, Andrew Slavin, Douglas Sawin, Susan Schrader, Jim Struve, and Louise Wisechild.

For help with the bibliography: Shana Ross, Jaimee Carroll, Barb Gore, Lynn Bryant, Susan Schrader, and Monica Gretter.

For the title, Shauna Smith.

Laura Hough for another beautiful design.

Personally, I'd like to thank:

The following friends and supporters: Kore Archer, George Brooks, Janet Bryer, Susan Bryer, Lauren Crux, Barbara Cymrot, Natalie Devora, Carol Anne Dwight, Steve Eckert, Harriet Elkington, Sue Estler, Laura Giges, Natalie Goldberg, Kay Hagan, Diane Hamer, Kate Hill, Leslie Ingram, Paula Johnson, Shama Khalethia, Aurora Levins Morales, Gilly McBlaze, Jennifer Meyer, Patrick Meyer, Leilani Miller, Robin Moulds, Nona Olivia, Barbara Ohrstrom, Jonathan Pannor, Celine Marie Pascale, Judy Phillips, Bryan Rawles, Paula Ross, Geneen Roth, Roberta Rutkin, Jan Simon, Jeanne Simonoff, Bert Simpson, Shauna Smith, Stephanie Smith, Matt Weinstein, Wendy Williams, and Dafna Wu.

My healers: Martha Benedict, Maya Clemis, Kathryn Lydecker, Jillellen McKee, Karen Sallowitz, and Dan Stickle for easing my pain and helping me stay in my body.

Ophelia Balderrama for taking care of Abe when I needed to write.

Ellen Bass for great feedback and friendship, and for making me dinner.

Karen Zelin for pulling me through some rough places.

Nona Olivia for inspiration, humor, good times, and friendship.

Barbara, Dafna, and Ruby for being part of my family.

Karyn Bristol for patience, persistence, and love.

Temme Davis for her courage, vitality, and willingness to grow.

Dear Reader:

I offer trainings for professionals, public lectures on healing from child sexual abuse, and workshops for partners. If you are interested in bringing me to your area, please contact my agent:

Denise Notzon
1450 Sixth Street
Berkeley, CA 94710

As a working writer, I regret that I am unable to answer individual letters, phone calls, or requests for referrals. (Contact the organizations listed in the resource section for referrals.) For reasons of confidentiality, I also cannot put you in contact with any of the people whose stories appear in "Partners' Stories." I do read my mail, however, and if you have feedback or responses to this book, I'd be happy to hear from you. If you want to be on my mailing list, send a note to the address below.

In the spirit of healing,

Laura Davis
P.O. Box 8503
Santa Cruz, CA 95061-8503

"This whole thing was new to me. I never knew much about incest."
—Mary, forty-six-year-old partner

"It's moved from being an unrecognized problem to a vaguely recognized problem to a present it's-here-all-the-time kind of situation. It's kind of grown into a monster."
—Eddie, thirty-four-year-old partner

"I've sat in bed and had these emotions churning and I've thought, 'I should know how to do this.' There's this guy out there who's the perfect partner. If I could just get into his brain, I'd do this partner thing right. You know the guy I'm talking about. He's the one who says, 'It's okay, honey, if we don't have sex for two years. I can do that.' I hated the guy."
—Jack, thirty-six-year-old partner

INTRODUCTION

In the last fifteen years, the sexual abuse of children has become an acknowledged social and political problem. Adults who were sexually abused as children have broken the silence, talked about their abuse, formed support groups, and courageously struggled to heal from the pain they've carried throughout their lives. There is a strong and powerful healing movement that offers resources, support, and advocacy to survivors of child sexual abuse.[1]

In the midst of this growing movement, there is one group that has been consistently overlooked—partners of survivors. Partners are people involved in intimate relationships with survivors—girlfriends, boyfriends, husbands, wives, and lovers. If you consider the statistics—that an estimated one in four girls and one in seven boys are sexually abused by the time they reach eighteen—and you think about the fact that most of these survivors grow up to form intimate relationships, it's clear your situation is not unique. There are partners of survivors everywhere.

Whether or not you were abused as a child yourself, the fact that you are involved in a relationship with a survivor means that

---

[1] Although survivors have made tremendous gains in the last fifteen years, it's important to acknowledge that there is a long way to go. Many survivors are still extremely isolated and resources remain poor in many areas. Most importantly, children are still being sexually abused in large numbers.

you, too, are living with the effects of abuse. Survivors frequently have difficulties with trust, commitment, sex, and intimacy, and these problems have a direct impact on you and your relationship.

This book will reassure you that it's possible to have a satisfying, mutual relationship with a survivor. It will encourage you to take care of yourself, teach you to look to your own needs, and show you how to support the survivor in your life without selling yourself short.

But you need more than words to support you. Books can be invaluable, but they don't give you someone to call in the middle of the night. Being the partner of a survivor can be lonely and frustrating at times, and you need people to support you when things get rough. I strongly encourage you to reach out by talking to a counselor, or a friend, or by starting a support group for partners. (See pages 39 and 162 for more on reaching out.)

WHERE AM I RIGHT NOW?

Listed below are some of the common reasons you might pick up this book. Feel free to check off the ones that apply to you:

_____ I'm about to make a commitment in a relationship. My girl-friend was sexually abused as a child.

_____ Everything was going fine until we got closer. Then things fell apart. I'm trying to find out why.

_____ I've just broken up with a survivor. I want to understand what happened.

_____ My husband doesn't want to make love anymore. I think it might have something to do with the things his brother did to him.

_____ I just started dating someone who was sexually abused. I wonder what kind of effect it's going to have on us.

_____ My lover has just "discovered" that he's an incest survivor. I'm skeptical. I want him to get over it so things can get back to normal.

_____ All the focus is on her and her memories. What about my needs?

_____ My boyfriend started going to therapy and suggested I read this.

_____ My lover doesn't remember anything from her childhood and is starting to get these funny feelings that something bad happened.

_____ Since this came up, I feel like I've been in a nightmare. When is it going to end?

_____ My girlfriend was raped by a couple of neighborhood boys when she was growing up. She says it didn't affect her, but I think it did.

_____ My husband is a survivor and he doesn't tell me much about what he's going through. I thought this book might help us communicate.

_____ My wife and I are doing pretty well now. We just need help with sex.

_____ I feel like I'm the only person in the world dealing with a spouse who's suicidal. I'm so scared. I don't know what to do.

_____ I'm thinking of leaving the relationship. This book is my last resort.

_____ My wife and I are both survivors. Things are nuts. We're like two three-year-olds half of the time. We need help.

_____ I'm not sure it's good for me to experience so much distance and deprivation. Should I stay or should I leave?

_____ I'm an alcoholic, and my lover was raped by her father. We're fighting all the time. I think it's her fault; she thinks it's mine.

_____ I'm a survivor, and my partner is starting to have memories. I'm not sure I want to go through it again.

_____ I'm a survivor, and I want to see things from my partner's viewpoint.

_____ I'm a survivor. I want to know what I'm going to face when I get in a relationship.

_____ I'm a counselor, and I'm looking for a resource I can use.

If you check off anything on the list, this book will have something to offer you. Keep reading. You'll find validation for your feelings, answers to many of your most pressing questions, and strategies for dealing with tough problems. You'll hear from dozens of other partners in your shoes. Their words will inspire you and reassure you that you're not alone.

WHOSE PROBLEMS ARE WE DEALING WITH?

Many of the problems addressed in this book are not unique to couples where one or both are survivors. Most couples struggle with issues of control, intimacy, trust, and sexuality. You're not having these problems solely because you're with a survivor. Everyone comes to relationships with baggage from their past, and although yours might not have to do with sexual abuse, it is there nonetheless. (See pages 56 and 143 for more on this important idea.)

Since the publication of *The Courage to Heal* in 1988, I've been traveling around the country talking to survivors, training counselors, and leading workshops for partners. At the beginning of each partners' workshop, I ask everyone an introductory set of questions:

"How many of you came from a home with at least one alcoholic parent?" "From a home where there was physical abuse?" "Emotional abuse or neglect?"

"How many of you lived with a mentally ill parent?" "Had a sibling who was sexually abused?" "Were sexually abused yourself?"

"How many of you are drug addicts or alcoholics?" "Are in a 12-step recovery program?" "Are war veterans with your own post-traumatic stress to deal with?"

Even though I give people permission not to raise their hands, hands go up all over the room. There's a lot of laughter and camaraderie as people look around. Many people raise their hands for more than one category. One man joked in the middle of this exercise, "Do I have to keep swinging my arm up and down? Can't I just keep my hand up for everything?"

I pause after the last question, and then say, "I have one more question to ask. How many people here came from a home they feel was basically healthy and happy?" Out of a hundred partners, usually ten raise their hands. (And by my estimation, five are probably in denial.)

You may be picking up this book because you want to understand more about sexual abuse and the impact it is having on your relationship. You may want to learn how to minimize those effects. You may want help with specific problem areas. You will get your answers. This book is full of them. But you will also be asked to shift your focus from the survivor and the survivor's problems to yourself —your needs, your feelings, your history, the places you can grow.

I was reading through some old workshop evaluations recently. At the bottom of his evaluation form, one man scrawled: "I made an observation today. The people who complained the most about the survivor's behavior were people who took the attitude that it was all the survivor's problem. The partners who were making it through the crisis were the ones who were willing to stand up and say they had problems and growing to do, too."

I couldn't agree more. As you read through the responses and stories in this book, keep an open mind. The best way for you and the survivor to make it through this process is to view it as a mutual journey.

ABOUT THIS BOOK

At the start of every partners' workshop, I ask each person to write their most pressing questions on an index card. The questions are always poignant and cut straight to the hart of things: "What percentage of survivors can be healed, and what is the average time period for healing?" "How can I stop being a nice guy and make sure my own needs get met?" "Will she love me in the end?" "How do I know when to throw in the towel?"

The first part of this book "Partners' Questions," answers these and other questions drawn directly from the partners' workshops.

As you read, you'll see that some of the answers are practical, offering suggestions, ideas, and strategies for coping with specific problems. Others are more philosophical; they ask you to examine your beliefs, values, and feelings. You'll also find a variety of exercises you and the survivor can do together.

The questions are grouped by category: The Basics, Allies in Healing, My Needs and Feelings, Dealing with Crisis, More about Sexual Abuse, Intimacy and Communication, Sex, Family Issues, and Final Thoughts. Flip through the book and look for the headings that interest you. You can begin anywhere. There may be sections you want to share with the survivor, and other parts you want to think through on your own. You can use this book in the way that best suits your needs.

It's important to note, however, that there are no definitive answers that hold true for every couple. Each survivor is at a different point in the healing process. Each partner has a unique history and set of needs. Where relationships are concerned, there are always more exceptions than rules. So while I can talk about ideal solutions, real life rarely fits the ideal. There is no one formula for having a successful relationship with a survivor, but the responses in this book can help you find answers that work for you.

The second part of this book, "Partners' Stories," explores the struggles, triumphs, and courage of eight partners. Their stories are important because of their diversity, and also because they give a human face to the concepts and ideas in this book.

Throughout the book, you'll see quotes and stories from partners. These are drawn from the hundreds of partners I've met in workshops, and from the twenty-five partners I interviewed in depth for this book. The interviews provided me with a wealth of material: I couldn't tell each person's story in its entirety, but I've included portions of each. Most of the quotes you'll see are unidentified; each one stands alone and represents one person's experience.

ABOUT LANGUAGE

Throughout this book, the word "partner" will be used instead of "wife," "husband," "spouse," or "lover" (except in the questions, where I've left the original language intact). Partner is a more inclusive word. It fits for all kinds of couples: married couples, unmarried couples, gay and lesbian couples.

The word "survivor" will be used to describe anyone who has survived child sexual abuse. I consciously use the word "survivor" instead of "victim" because it communicates a feeling of empowerment and possibility.

I've varied my use of pronouns throughout the book since both men and women are sexually abused, both men and women are partners, and both men and women abuse children. Focus on yourself and the particulars of your situation, changing pronouns as needed. That way, the shifts from "he" to "she" shouldn't leave you feeling left out.

IF YOU ARE A SURVIVOR READING THIS BOOK . . .

Even though this book was written for partners, there is also a lot you can learn from it. It's full of information about sexual abuse, strategies for coping with problem areas, guidelines for forming a healthier relationship, and exercises you can do with your partner. If you're in a relationship, you might want to read it together. (If you're not ready to read it at all, or only want to read the sections your partner asks you to, that's fine too.)

Remember, however, that this book was written with the needs of partners in mind. It does not teach partners to be perfectly supportive of the survivors in their lives. Rather, it teaches them to look at themselves, pay attention to their own feelings, assert their own needs, and take care of themselves. This may or may not lead to you getting the kind of support you want or hope for.

There may be times this book will be hard for you to read. It talks a lot about the difficulties of being involved with a survivor. You will hear from partners who are angry, sick of being supportive, and tired of hearing about sexual abuse. You will meet partners who have left their relationships, or are thinking of leaving. You'll also read stories that are hopeful and inspiring. At times, you may find yourself despairing about the relationship you're in, or worrying that no one will ever love you.

I'd like to encourage you to assume the attitude I ask survivors to take when they sit in on a partners' workshop. As much as you can, put aside your own needs, feelings, and desires. Think of yourself as an observer who is getting the chance to learn about things from a partner's perspective. See this as an opportunity to step out of yourself and see that partners hurt too.

When you're healing from sexual abuse, it's easy to become self-absorbed; to forget that the abuse is affecting not just you but also the people you love the most. Knowing that you're not the only one whose life has been turned upside-down is a necessary step toward becoming real allies. See if you can use this book as a way to listen. Let it form the basis of a more honest dialogue with your partner.

PART I:
PARTNERS' QUESTIONS

THE BASICS

"This has been the year of sexual abuse. Once it started opening up, it's been everywhere around me."

"I have to keep reminding myself, 'This isn't personal. This is what happens when someone is healing from child sexual abuse.'"

"There's a part of me that would like to have a wife who has it all together. I'd come home and she would be there, looking all refreshed, carrying a tray of cookies and milk. Instead, she comes out, looking bedraggled, and has a memory to tell me about. She's not June Cleaver."

"It's just too big to go 'poof' and make it better."

What is child sexual abuse?

Child sexual abuse is a violation of power perpetrated by a person with more power over someone who is more vulnerable. This violation takes a sexual form, but it involves more than sex. It involves a breach of trust, a breaking of boundaries, and a profound violation of the survivor's sense of self. It is a devastating and selfish crime.

The most important thing in defining child sexual abuse is the experience of the child. It takes very little for a child's world to be devastated. A single experience can have a profound impact on a child's life. A man sticks his hand in his daughter's underpants, or strokes his son's penis once, and for that child, the world is never the same again. As a partner, it's crucial that you believe the survivor and learn about the impact abuse can have.

Child sexual abuse includes a broad range of experiences. Girls and boys are abused by fathers, mothers, stepparents, uncles, aunts, cousins, siblings, grandparents, family friends, foster parents, neighbors, teachers, Little League coaches, rabbis, ministers, religious counselors, psychiatrists and other doctors, therapists, police officers, camp counselors, neighborhood kids, and strangers. Sexual abuse can begin in infancy, childhood, or adolescence. It can be a one-time experience or something which happens repeatedly.

Some abuse is of a covert nature and doesn't involve physical touch. A young girl is developing breasts and as she dresses in the morning, her father watches with a sexual interest, making lewd comments about her body. A young boy tries to go to the bathroom, but his mother is always in the room, asking the boy if he masturbates and how. A football coach insists on seeing his players naked before they can make the team. He makes crude, suggestive remarks about their penises. These are examples of abuse where the perpetrator does not physically touch the child. But they are traumatic nonetheless.

Children are fondled, raped, french kissed, forced to perform fellatio and cunnilingus, forced to watch sexual acts, and made to have sex with each other. Sometimes abuse is couched in "gentle" cuddling or touches; other times it is violent, coupled with beatings or torture. Ritual abuse, a particularly horrifying form of abuse, involves severe physical, sexual, and psychological abuse of children by organized groups of perpetrators. (For more on ritual and cult abuse, see page 132.)

Children both hate and love their abusers.

If you're not familiar with some of the horrible crimes perpetrated against children, you may find it hard to believe these things. Part of working with survivors (for me) and living with a survivor (for you) is that we have to accept the fact that human beings are capable of such atrocities.

If you haven't been abused yourself, particularly if you grew up in a "good" home, it may be difficult for you to believe that people molest, torture, and sexually abuse children. It may take time for you to fully accept the survivor's experience. Yet it is a powerful thing to do. Being intimately involved with a survivor makes you take in more of the world. When you let yourself feel and really see the sickness in the world, you also see more of its beauty. You no longer live on the surface. You have to go deep. When you're involved with someone who is fighting back and healing from abuse, you join in a struggle that says yes to life. As one partner told me, "If it hadn't been for this, I never would have woken up."

How is it going to affect me to be involved with a survivor?

To answer that question, you have to consider two things: where you are in your relationship and where the survivor is in terms of dealing with the abuse. If you're already in a long-term committed relationship with a survivor, and he's just beginning to look at issues of childhood sexual abuse, you're in a very different position than someone who's starting a brand-new relationship. Generally, the longer you've been together and the more history and commitment you've built, the better equipped you'll be to deal with the stresses involved in facing the abuse. That's not to say a new relationship with a survivor can't work out; it's just that it's usually harder— there's less of an investment in the relationship to back you up when things get tough.

If the survivor in your life is just starting to deal with the abuse, you're probably facing years of fairly volatile change. Healing is slow, and the beginning is often the hardest. If, on the other hand, you're with a survivor who's been dealing with these issues for years, you'll be able to benefit from the growth and clarity he's already achieved.

No two survivors are alike, and only you know the inside of your particular relationship. One thing is clear, however. The more open you are to the idea of a relationship being a place in which to challenge yourself and grow, the more successful you'll be at being involved with a survivor. (For more on coping with change in relationships, see page 48.)

What are the most important characteristics for a partner of a survivor to possess?

Compassion, flexibility, resourcefulness, patience, humor, and knowledge of your own needs and limits.

When you're intimate with someone who has been sexually abused, it's natural to empathize with the pain, the anger, the feelings of shame and sadness; to feel outrage at the unfairness of the abuse. Compassion is the ability to enter someone else's world, to be touched by their pain without being consumed by it. Loving a survivor means that you love someone whose suffering you cannot control and will never fully know.

Life is often topsy-turvy when a survivor begins the healing process: you need to roll with the changes, adjust your expectations, and find new ways to meet your own neglected needs. That's where flexibility and resourcefulness come in.

Healing is slow, and the changes never seem quick enough. If you can develop an attitude of patience, while continuing to affirm your own needs and desires for your relationship, you will offer the survivor support without selling yourself short.

Humor is a necessary antidote to the heaviness of healing. Encourage the survivor to laugh, to take breaks, to have fun. If that's impossible, find small pockets of pleasure for yourself.

You also need to know your own limits. Not everyone wants to be in an intimate relationship with someone struggling to heal from child sexual abuse. Give yourself permission to leave or to consider leaving. That way, if you stay, your commitment will resonate with the power of free choice. (See page 87 for more on the decision to stay or go.)

How does sexual abuse affect children once they grow up?

Sexual abuse has severe long-term effects. It's important that you learn about these effects so you can better understand the impact they're having on both you and the survivor. Exploring the ways abuse affects your relationship might ease some of the confusion you're feeling right now. This isn't to say that all the problems you're facing are due to the fact that your partner was sexually abused as a child. You, too, bring a lifetime of history to your relationship. (For more on this, see page 56.)

Sexual abuse does not happen in a vacuum but in combination with other life experiences. The duration of the abuse, its severity, the closeness of the child to the offender, the dynamics of the family, and the presence or absence of support for the child all have a role in determining the later effects of abuse. In families where children are supported, listened to, and protected, the effects of the abuse in adulthood can be negligible. When children are discounted or further abused, the damage is made worse.

Other life factors (dealing with racism, divorce, poverty, war, disability, being an only child) and other forms of dysfunction (alcoholism, neglect, or physical abuse) all play a part in determining the way sexual abuse affects a particular child. For one child, sexual abuse is the most pervasive influence in their lives; for others, the death of a parent is much more significant. In some families, the effects of alcoholism, violence, and sexual abuse blur together.

As you learn about the effects of abuse, you will find some fit the survivor in your life, and others don't. The survivor may be highly functional at work, but have a lot of trouble with intimacy; may be good at communication and parenting, but have problems with sex. Or she might be having trouble with everything. One partner explained, "Incest gets into every aspect of the relationship. I like to heat the plates before dinner, which seems to be a semi-normal thing to do. We've had fights about it because her perpetrator did that. She says, 'I can't *stand* it when someone warms the plates.'"

As you learn about the long-term effects of abuse, you may feel helpless, frustrated, or depressed by the recognition that so many of the struggles you face as a couple echo back to the abuse. Take your time as you read through the next few pages. If you're not familiar with the dynamics of sexual abuse, you may be shocked at how much of an influence they have had on your own life. Pay particular attention to the sections on intimate relationships and sexuality. These are likely to be the areas in which the survivor's history will have the greatest impact on you.

SELF-ESTEEM

What Happens in Childhood

The child's boundaries are violated. He loses any sense of control and gets the message he's not valued. He's humiliated and his real needs are ignored. He's isolated from family members and peers. In many cases, the child is blamed for the abuse, told he's crazy or making up lies. The child's reality and sense of the world are greatly distorted.

What This Means in Adulthood

Adult survivors believe the abuse was their fault, that they're not worth much, and that somehow they're different than other people. Survivors say things like: "It's as if everyone else is on the other side of this glass wall living real, normal lives. And I'm over here on this side of the glass all by myself. I feel like I'm from another planet." Or, "If you ever really knew me, you wouldn't want to know me." The survivor often feels there's something bad, wrong, or dirty at his core. The sense of shame and self-loathing survivors feel is often hidden, but extremely deep. This self-hate is often expressed in two ways: the survivor tries to be perfect or good on the outside to make up for bad feelings on the inside and/or he acts out self-destructive feelings through suicidal feelings or suicide attempts, intentional self-injury, overindulgence in drugs, food, alcohol, unsafe sex or seeking out dangerous people or situations. Self-hate also shows up in more subtle ways. The survivor sabotages himself right before he achieves success or makes a commitment to a healthy relationship.

The survivor may also not know how to protect himself, how to pay attention to his own instincts, feelings, or inner voice. He doesn't believe he deserves to be treated with respect or caring. The predominant feeling in his life is one of powerlessness. This can lead him into dangerous situations or associations with people who hurt him further.

FEELINGS

What Happens in Childhood

Abuse manipulates and twists a child's natural sense of trust and love. Her innocent feelings are belittled or mocked, and she learns to ignore her feelings. She can't afford to feel the full range of feelings in her body while she's being abused—pain, outrage, hate, vengeance, confusion, arousal. So she short-circuits them and goes numb. For many children, any expression of feelings, even a single tear, is cause for more severe abuse. Again, the only recourse is to shut down. Feelings go underground.

What This Means in Adulthood

Adult survivors are often unaware of their feelings or only express feelings inappropriately. They get stuck on a particular emotion (like anger or sadness) and are unable to feel anything else. Because they don't value their feelings, they say things like "I wouldn't know a feeling if I fell over one," or "Feelings? They're such a bother." Emotions become scary and the survivor worries about losing control: "If I ever let myself get angry, I'd kill someone." "If I ever let myself cry, I'd never stop crying."

Yet we all have feelings. Whether we're aware of them or not, they exist. When survivors repress their feelings, they experience depression, nightmares, panic attacks, and sometimes become abusive themselves.

For many survivors, "good" feelings—contentment, happiness, pleasure, joy—are particularly frightening. Whenever things were calm or felt good at home as a child, disaster was sure to follow.

BODY AWARENESS

What Happens in Childhood

When a child is abused, the conflicting sensations he experiences (pain, anger, humiliation, arousal) are too much for him. Rather than give the abuser the satisfaction of seeing his body react, the child shuts down and "leaves" his body. As a result, survivors often describe their abuse as if they're watching a movie: "It was like I was up on the ceiling looking down at these things happening to some other child. I couldn't feel a thing."

What This Means in Adulthood

As adults, survivors are often extremely disconnected from their bodies, living only "from the neck up." "I thought of myself as a giant brain," one woman told me. "Body?" one man asked. "What body?" Many survivors hate their bodies and either ignore or abuse them. Others compensate for the "betrayal of their body" through excessive working out, weight training, and exercise, in an attempt to make their bodies so strong that no one can ever hurt them again.

Dissociation (splitting off from the self) becomes automatic for many survivors. When he's upset, threatened, or sexually aroused, the survivor checks out. When this happens, you get the eerie feeling that you're with him but really all alone. It's almost as if no one is at home. No one is. The survivor has taken his attention away. Only his body is left behind. (For more on the continuum of dissociation, see page 136.)

INTIMACY

What Happens in Childhood

Abused children receive confusing messages about sex and love, trust and betrayal. The abuser often says, "I'm doing this because I love you," and then proceeds to hurt the child. The child learns she can't trust the people she loves, and that she doesn't have a choice about being close to someone else; people take what they want, regardless. Love becomes a dangerous force, wrought with confusion, pain, and violation.

What This Means in Adulthood

Most adult survivors struggle with the issue of trust—either trusting inappropriately or not trusting at all. Many are severely isolated and scared of being close. Relationships that combine love and sex are fraught with confusion and dangers. Instead of love feeling like love—safe, warm, and positive—for the survivor, it feels like potential annihilation. When you say "I love you" to a survivor, you can never be sure of the response you're going to get.

Survivors often develop an exaggerated need for control in their adult relationships. It's the only way they feel safe. They also struggle with commitment—saying yes in a relationship means being trapped in yet another family situation where abuse might take place. So the survivor panics as your relationship gets closer, certain that something terrible is going to happen. She pulls away, rejects you, or tests you all the time. (For more, see "Intimacy and Communication" on page 142.)

SEXUALITY

What Happens in Childhood

When a child is sexually abused, his normal sexual development is cut short. He's forced to be sexual on an adult's timetable. He doesn't get to feel his own desire, sexual orientation, or interest. Nor does he get the chance to explore sex in an age-appropriate way. He learns that desire (the abuser's desire, is a scary, out-of-control force. The child's first experiences of sexual arousal are linked with shame, disgust, pain, and humiliation. This makes for powerful imprinting. If the abuse was linked with affection and nurturing, the child grows up confused about the difference between affection and sex, intimacy and intrusion.

What This Means in Adulthood

Many survivors are celibate, choose partners who don't want sex, or find other creative ways to avoid having a full sexual life. Survivors are often scared of sex, think it's basically "dirty," or see it as an obligation they must perform. The survivor forces himself to "go through the motions," even though he's numb, absent, or in a panic.

Violent or abusive fantasies may arouse the survivor, and this can cause deep shame. Other times, he may experience flashbacks to the abuse, in which he can't differentiate between you, his partner today, and the abuser. Sex becomes a mine field full of painful associations and memories.

Other survivors act out sexually and become promiscuous. The survivor was told he was only good for sex, and he fulfills that legacy, sometimes with a disregard for his own safety. His sense of well-being and self-esteem gets hooked up with sexual desirability. Sex becomes the primary way he feels connected and cared for. Never having learned how to say no to sex, he takes the position, "If someone wants me, of course I have sex with them." Sex becomes a source of power, a way to manipulate, to gain control. (For more on sexual issues, see "Sex" on page 176.)

THE SURVIVOR'S FAMILY

What Happens in Childhood

Incest and sexual abuse take place in an environment of secrecy, lies, and silence. When abuse takes place within a family, the child learns that her family is a dangerous place where people hurt each other. She learns that her parents will not protect her, and in fact, may be the source of her pain. Usually, she is isolated from other family members, and her peers as well. Often she is blamed for her family's troubles.

What This Means in Adulthood

If the survivor's abuse took place in her family, relationships with her family are likely to be strained. The essential mistrust, silence, and abuse of power that existed in her family are probably still there. The abuse may still be a secret and the abuser may still be at it: ruining the lives of the next generation. This means, quite literally, that your children may be at risk. (See page 224 for a clearer warning about the dangers.)

The survivor is unlikely to get support from her family in dealing with abuse that took place within the family. She may be the family scapegoat, rejected or blamed for the problems in the family. This may leave her feeling crazy, depressed, or invalidated when she has contact with her family. (For more on family issues, see page 211.)

PARENTING

What Happens in Childhood

When a child is abused in his own home, he lacks positive role models for parenting. Instead, he sees parenting that is punitive, harsh, and often abusive. Often he is told he is doomed to repeat the cycle of abuse.

What This Means in Adulthood

Because of the prevalent (and false) myth that all abused children go on to abuse children, many survivors are afraid to become parents. When survivors haven't faced their own abuse, they sometimes abuse or fail to protect their own children. Most survivor-parents, however, become fierce protectors. Like the rest of us, survivors can make conscious, often painful efforts to be better parents: learning to set healthy boundaries and limits, communicate respectfully, and build their children's self-esteem. It's harder to do these things when no one did them for you, yet many survivors overcome the limitations of their parents and do a better job with their own children. (See page 234 for more on Parenting.)

WORK

What Happens in Childhood

A child who is being abused has little time to explore her interests or talents. Her education is often spotty. In her family, she is isolated and left to cope on her own; she has little chance to learn about cooperation and working as part of a team.

What This Means in Adulthood

Many adult survivors are confused about the kind of work they want to do. The survivor may have unrealistic job goals or keep trying to fulfill her family's ideas about the work she should (or shouldn't) be doing. Suffering from a lack of self-confidence, the survivor may have trouble making decisions and may consistently settle for less than she's capable of.

The workplace often mirrors family life; many survivors end up in jobs where the dynamics are similar to their families of origin. This can translate into difficulties with co-workers, personality conflicts, problems with bosses and other authority figures, or an overall feeling of being trapped. Survivors on the job are particularly prone to exploitation.

Some survivors use achievement as a way to compensate for deep feelings of inadequacy. The survivor's skills at controlling things and solving problems help her to succeed in the workplace.

She works harder than anyone else; no task is too difficult. She becomes a prized worker and a workaholic. The rest of her life suffers accordingly.

As you've read through this list of effects, you may have grown increasingly overwhelmed. Or you may feel relieved, because so much more of your experience with the survivor makes sense. You may feel angry about the abuse or feel hopeless at the enormity of the problem.

You may have also recognized some of the effects of abuse in your own life. If you were neglected or abused as a child, you may be realizing that those early experiences had more of an effect on you than you previously thought. Other kinds of traumas (war, for instance) can produce many of the effects listed above; but you may also find yourself wondering if there's something from your past you've overlooked or forgotten. (See page 56 for more on exploring your own history).

If both you and your partner have been abused, you may have seen both similarities and differences in the ways the abuse affected you. The places your problems dovetail are probably the places you'll experience the most conflict and the greatest potential for growth. (See "Survivor-Survivor Relationships" on page 58 for more.)

The most important thing to say about the effects of abuse is that most of them can be reversed or mitigated to a large degree. Overcoming the limiting effects of abuse is one of the primary reasons the survivor is facing the abuse to begin with. With a solid commitment to healing and good support, tremendous change is possible. The effects of abuse do not have to last forever.

What percentage of survivors can be healed, and what is the average time period for healing?

Under proper conditions, one hundred percent of survivors can heal. Survivors are like seedlings. With proper conditions—light, air, warmth, food, and water—plants grow. Survivors are the same way. When their desire to heal is met with information, skilled support, and a safe environment, they begin to grow in ways they never dreamed possible. The sad thing is that not all survivors have access to these conditions. Many are still being abused, don't have access to information or support, and are still terribly isolated. Some have tried to get help only to be reabused by the people who were supposed to be there to help them. Others don't want to change or don't believe they can. Hopefully, resources and information will continue to grow, services will become increasingly affordable, and more and more survivors will be in a position where they have the support necessary to heal.

I could not work with survivors if I thought that the damage from child sexual abuse was irreparable. I deeply believe that survivors can overcome the damage of abuse. It's difficult and slow, but it's possible.

"How long?" is one of the most heartfelt questions I hear. Survivors want to know, and you want to know, too: "How much longer do I have to live this way? If I hang in here, will it be worth it to me? Will there be a time when I will get more of what I need in this relationship? Is there hope for the person I love?"

The only answer I can give to the question "How long?" is that healing takes a long time. If you're with someone who's commited and active in her healing, things will continue to change, and over time, improve. But there is no time frame I can give you. I can't say, "Well, this crisis period will last another year and then she'll be ready to deal with sex." I can only say that very little will stay the same for long. You won't be dealing with the same crisis in the same way two years from now. You may be facing a different kind of crisis, or the same kind of crisis with better strategies, or you may be experiencing a period of calm and closeness where abuse has faded from center stage. It's hard to predict. Sometimes things get worse before they get better, but if you hang in there over the long haul, gradually they change for the better. Life begins to be about all of life, not just about the impediments.

People always ask me, "Are you healed?" I can't answer yes to that question because I don't believe there's a finish line. But I do know if I sat down and read the voluminous journals I kept during the first couple of years after I remembered my abuse, it would be like reading about someone else's life. I would find little resemblance between the suffering I was experiencing then to my life today. The immensity of my pain and my need to focus on it exclusively would be hard for me to relate to. I would vaguely remember feeling that way, I would be able to say, "Yes, I needed to do that," but the pain itself would seem kind of dim and far away. I'm glad. Healing was a way to get through the pain to something else. I didn't want to hurt forever. I wanted to move on—and I have.

Healing is definitely possible. Seven years ago, when things were at their worst for me, there were times I wanted to give up or wished I was dead. As far as I could tell, my life was always going to be this way. Pain created more pain. I couldn't see a way out. I remember thinking I would never have a moment when I wasn't absorbed in child sexual abuse, obsessed with my own healing, or yanked out of the present to remember some atrocity.

I was wrong. I have a life now. It's not a perfect life, but it's a good one. It has integrity and joy and moments of real pleasure. I'm not always happy, but I am rooted in the present. I'm no longer sentenced to play out the past, over and over again. It's been worth it to heal. It continues to be worth it.

I've accepted the fact that I will be dealing with issues connected to my abuse for the rest of my life. Not always, but sometimes. When I take on a new challenge or go deeper with someone I love, I will see new wrinkles, new ways that the abuse tore at my spirit. But I have the skills, knowledge, and support to deal with it. It doesn't have to stop my life. Abuse no longer diminishes me or robs me of my right to a life in the present. I'm not damaged; I'm a whole person.

Any survivor can make it to this place. There is nothing extraordinary about me that doesn't exist in every other human being. I had the desire. I was lucky enough to get the support. I made the commitment and I followed through. It's taken years, but it's been worth it.

HOW LONG DOES IT TAKE TO HEAL?

As a partner, you can provide a backbone of support and safety for the survivor you love. You can hold out the belief that it's possible. If the rest of us do our part—making support services for survivors affordable, accessible, and widespread—the pieces will be in place. Healing will become an empowering revolution and not just a privilege of the few.

What does it take to overcome the effects of abuse?

Healing takes hard work, determination, and time. Although every survivor heals in a different way, there are certain common stages survivors go through as they work to overcome the effects of abuse in their lives. These stages make up "the healing process."[1]

The healing process is best described as a spiral. Survivors go through the stages once, sometimes many times; sometimes in one order, sometimes in another. Each time they hit a stage again, they move up the spiral: they can integrate new information and a broader range of feelings, utilize more resources, take better care of themselves, and make deeper changes.

THE DECISION TO HEAL

The survivor is ready to face the abuse and explore the impact it's had on her life. She makes an active commitment to heal: to find help, seek the truth, face the unknown, make changes, and feel the feelings necessary to resolve the pain. She renews this commitment again and again as she faces new challenges and deeper levels of pain.

Being with a survivor who's made the decision to heal means you'll be dealing with sexual abuse for some time in your relationship. Keep reading. You'll learn more about what you can expect and what you'll need to do to take care of yourself.

THE EMERGENCY STAGE

When a survivor first remembers his abuse or decides to heal, he often (but not always) goes through the emergency stage, a period of crisis in which he, and often you by extension, is immersed in

---

[1] These stages were first outlined by Ellen Bass and me in *The Courage to Heal.*

dealing with sexual abuse. The characteristics of the emergency stage (length, intensity, kinds of crisis) vary from survivor to survivor, but the core of it is this: the survivor is obsessed with sexual abuse and finds it difficult to think, talk, or pay attention to anything else.

The survivor's task during the emergency stage is to gradually integrate the terrible reality that he was sexually abused. Survivors are frequently bombarded with memories, uncontrollable feelings, and deep, wrenching pain. They're reliving the painful feelings and sensations they felt at the time they were abused. The intensity of the experience overshadows everything else in their lives. Survivors often have trouble working, living, even taking care of themselves on the most basic level during the emergency stage. They may act out self-destructive urges or feel suicidal. As a partner, dealing with a survivor in the emergency stage can be terrifying. Turn to page 91 for help dealing with times of crisis.

REMEMBERING

Some survivors have always remembered what happened to them; others begin to suspect later in their lives that they were abused. For survivors who've always remembered the abuse, remembering involves delving into the feelings they had, looking at the effects, and acknowledging the damage in their lives. For survivors who forgot the abuse entirely, remembering involves putting together recollections, bits of memory, body sensations, physical responses to other people's stories, conversations with family members, and other clues to get a sense of the abuse. Some survivors go through periods of intense flashbacks, where they relive and rewitness aspects of the abuse. Others never recover clear memories, but nonetheless, find ways to piece the puzzle together.

As a partner, you may be deeply involved in the survivor's process of recovering memories (see "Noah's Story" on page 258) or you may choose to stay more separate (see "Virginia's Story" on page 293). But however you work things out with the survivor, you will still be affected. Her pain, anguish, and grief at remembering will spill out onto your life together. (For more on memories and flashbacks, see pages 115, 118, and 187.)

BELIEVING IT HAPPENED

Many survivors struggle to believe the abuse happened. They don't want to believe it. It's too painful to think about. They don't want to accuse family members or face the terrible loss involved in realizing "a loved one" hurt them; they don't want to rock the boat. Many survivors were told they were crazy or liars for so long, they don't trust themselves. "I must be making this up," one man said. "I always did have a vivid imagination." Others struggle to believe the abuse took place because their memories are sketchy or incomplete. For all of these reasons, it is difficult for survivors to consistently accept and believe that the abuse took place.

Often, the survivor's ability to hold his belief comes and goes. Ellen Bass describes it like this: "When the survivor believes the abuse, he feels pain, terror, and anguish. When he doesn't believe it, he feels intense self-hatred for 'making it up.' He often flips back and forth between the two, until, eventually, the pain of dealing with the abuse becomes preferable to the intense feelings of self-hate."

Survivors aren't the only ones who struggle to believe the abuse took place. Partners often have a hard time grappling with the reality of abuse. If you're having trouble believing the survivor, turn to page 51 for more on handling these feelings.

BREAKING SILENCE

Abuse takes place in an environment of secrecy and silence. In order to heal, it's critical for survivors to talk about their abuse. The survivor can tell one person or a thousand, but the crucial thing is for her to let the secret out and to share the truth of her experience with at least one caring, loving, responsive listener. Otherwise, she continues to live with the horror of the experience alone.

Breaking silence can involve finding a therapist, joining a support group, telling friends, or letting you know about her childhood experiences. Initially, telling is scary; many survivors say things like "I'll die if I tell," or "She'll come and get me if I tell." After a while, though, survivors become more comfortable talking about the abuse. Sometimes, in fact, they go through a stage where they want to tell everyone. I did that for a time: "Hello, my name is Laura Davis. I'm happy to meet you and did you know I was an incest survivor?"

For some survivors, breaking silence becomes more than just a personal step in their healing journey. It becomes a political commitment. They choose to speak out publicly as a way of fighting back against abuse. Survivors have organized art shows, rallies, marches, speak-outs, conferences, media events, and information networks. These are all empowering, effective ways of breaking the silence.

As a partner, you will have to confront your own beliefs about speaking out, "airing dirty laundry," saying things that "aren't nice." You will also have to decide whether you want people to know that you are the partner of a survivor. (See page 162 for a discussion of this sensitive issue.)

UNDERSTANDING IT WASN'T THEIR FAULT

Almost universally, children believe they are to blame for the abuse. They think there is some bad seed, some shameful, dirty, bad part of them that caused the abuse to occur. Abusers plant and reinforce these beliefs; children are trusting and believe them.

Children can't afford to see the adults around them as bad: as long as the survivor believed he was somehow at fault ("I needed the attention, wanted the affection, took the candy, rode the bicycle, loved the abuser, had an orgasm"), he could hold on to the false hope that he could stop the abuse by changing his behavior. This belief, although twisted and self-defeating, is more bearable to a child than seeing his caretakers as violent or hurtful.

Many adult survivors still believe that the abuse was their fault. One of the main tasks of healing is understanding, not just intellectually but at a gut level, that the abuse was the abuser's fault; that no matter what the survivor did, felt, said, or didn't do as a child (or a teenager or a young adult), he wasn't to blame.

To be a supportive partner, you'll need to accept this basic truth as well: No matter what the circumstances, abuse is always the fault of the abuser.

GETTING IN TOUCH WITH THE INNER CHILD

Most survivors grew up too fast; their more vulnerable child-selves got lost in the need to protect and deaden themselves. Reclaiming the inner child is part of the healing process. Often the inner child holds information and feelings for the adult; when the adult makes contact with the child, she's able to recover memories and feelings that have been buried for a lifetime. Some of these feelings are painful; others are actually fun. The child holds the playfulness and innocence the adult has had to bury. Integrating the child-self brings a fuller, richer life.

To a partner, this integration of the inner child can be baffling at times. If you find yourself missing the grown-up you thought you were involved with, see page 102.

GRIEVING AND MOURNING

Integrating feelings is another crucial part of the healing process. As the survivor begins to realize the extent of the damage and begins to tally his losses, he's going to experience tremendous grief. Grieving for the tragedy of child sexual abuse is similar to grieving for other kinds of loss. Survivors need to grieve for their lost childhoods, stolen innocence, missed opportunities, lack of family, the state of the world, today's child victims, and a thousand other losses. Since many survivors have been numb and closed to their feelings, this period of grieving is often marked by an outpouring of tears, many of which have been buried for years.

As a partner, you will have your own grieving to do. A lot of what's been known and familiar to you is shifting and there's no guarantee as to how things will end up. You will grieve with the survivor, but also for your own losses: changed relationships with in-laws, loss of ease around sex, the survivor's preoccupation with abuse, the cost in money and time that healing requires. Your specific losses will vary, depending on you and your relationship, but it's inevitable that you will have your own mourning to do.

ANGER

Anger is the backbone of healing. Most survivors have been angry for years. Either they've turned it in on themselves or lashed out at others and become abusive themselves. As a survivor heals, she learns to direct her anger clearly and squarely at the abuser and the people who failed to protect her. The survivor needs to find safe, empowering ways to express her anger and let it out. This can include physical releases (hitting softballs, pounding on pillows, running), taking action in the world (channeling the anger into activism), or confronting the abuser.

As a partner, you will be angry too: your life is changing, your needs aren't being met, you have to spend all this time dealing with a problem you didn't create. It's easy to direct all this anger at the survivor. See if you can focus it on the abuser instead. (See pages 79 and 99 for more on dealing with anger.)

CONFRONTING THE ABUSER

Confronting the abuser is a powerful way to express anger and affirm the truth. Confronting the offender can be a way to let go, to move on, to give up unrealistic fantasies of reconciliation. Although not all survivors choose to confront directly, doing so can be a critical step in healing. As much as possible, survivors should think things through and be prepared before the confrontation takes place.

If the survivor in your life wants to confront the abuser or members of his family, your beliefs about speaking out and "making trouble" will be challenged. Also, confrontations are one of the areas in which you, as a partner, can offer the most practical support. (For suggestions on ways you can help, see page 216.)

RESOLUTION AND MOVING ON

After moving through these stages several times, the survivor eventually reaches the stage of resolution and moving on. This is what you've been waiting for: the major tasks of healing have been accomplished, the obsession with abuse diminishes, and life in the present comes back into focus. Instead of looking backwards toward the abuser and the abuse, the survivor is increasingly able to focus on her life today as an adult. The resolution stage is one of integration. Things stabilize. The survivor is able to make lasting changes in areas such as intimacy, sexuality, work, and parenting. Her attention is on the present and the ways you both can grow, individually and in your relationship. (For more on the stage of resolution and moving on, see page 238.)

Survivors who've moved through the stages of the healing process are weathered and resilient. They know how to make a commitment and to follow something through. They've gained confidence in their ability to face terrible trials; and they've learned more about the preciousness of life. Survivors who've reached the stage of moving on have a greater capacity for compassion, caring, and living fully. If you're able to see the process through together, your relationship will have been strengthened and enriched beyond measure. When you get to the place where you can look back and say, "Wow, we made it," you'll have proven beyond a doubt your stamina, creativity, commitment, and love.

Is the survivor aware of her partner's pain?

If the survivor in your life has just begun to heal, it's likely that you feel confused, angry, displaced, needy, and frightened. Something out of your control has come into your life and disrupted your home, your relationship, and your family. It's a disorienting time and there may be long stretches when you feel incidental to the monumental forces that are reshaping the survivor's life. For the most part this is true. The healing crisis is happening in her life, and is emanating out from there. You can be a supporter or a companion, but it's really her journey. You can choose to go with her, to explore the hidden (or not so hidden) pockets of pain in your own life, to use this crisis as an opportunity to grow, but don't expect much support from her in exchange. Often it's a long time before the survivor can look up, see your pain, and say, "Oh! Someone I love is hurting too. This is not just about me." As one partner put it, "With a survivor in crisis, there's a period when they're just not there for themselves, much less for anyone else."

There may be times when the survivor can't listen to anything about your life, not even for half an hour, when her obsession with the abuse is total and complete. Fortunately, this is not a stage that lasts forever, but when she is in the middle of it, you may feel lonelier than you've ever felt. As one partner put it, "If you have a fear of abandonment, you'd better start dealing with it now."

When I talk to survivors, I tell them that no matter how self-absorbed they are, they still have to give something back if they're in a relationship. Even if it's ten minutes of attention a week, just saying, "I know you have feelings too. And someday, I want to be able to pay attention." They need to offer something. In a period of extreme crisis, even this may be impossible, but it's unfair for the survivor to take the attitude "You exist to support me; you should just bury your own feelings and needs." This is unrealistic. You are human too. You have problems of your own, and now the survivor's pain is having a profound impact on your life.

Through the survivor's self-absorption (which may be necessary for her), you will be forced to become independent in ways you may have never considered. As one partner put it, "You've got to have other friends, because there are times when the survivor will be completely in her own world, and you won't be able to share anything with her."

This is a not a time when the two of you can be a self-sufficient unit, meeting each other's every desire and need. You can either shift your expectations or walk around angry, resentful, and unfulfilled. You will need to become more resourceful, to get more support from other people, to find new ways to feel good about who you are and what you need. (For practical help with this, try working through the exercises on pages 75 and 169.)

In time, the survivor has to learn to consider you too, but it may take years before your relationship exists in a real equilibrium. In the meantime, you have to learn to live with things the way they are. As one partner put it so well:

> For the first six months after she remembered, I just kind of held my breath, waiting for it to be over. After half a year went by, I realized that I couldn't hold my breath forever. I couldn't continue to make myself that small and insignificant. I couldn't put myself on hold forever. I had to start breathing. I had to learn to live with it.

Learning to live with it is a painful, lonely challenge. If you're not flexible, if you can't stretch, if you can't let go of your life as it was before and accept the way it is now, you will be fighting every inch of the way. It's important for you to express your frustration and anger, but ultimately you have to make peace with what is. The survivor is not going to change back into the person she was before. You're no longer going to be naive and innocent about the terrible crimes that are committed in families in the name of love. You're not going to be able to look her mother in the face without thinking of the terrible things she did to her little girl. You're not going to stop waking up at night wondering if someone will get to your children as they walk to school, go to day-care, approach the world with fearlessness and wonder. Your innocence has been broken too, and nothing in your world will be the same. That's what being a partner is about.

In the beginning, the survivor will not be able to pick her head up long enough to realize you, too, have been changed, that your world has also been shattered and that you are grieving. It's important to find others in your situation. They will let you know you're not alone, that your pain matters too.

Is there anyone else here from Duluth?

Yes, there are partners of survivors everywhere. The difficulty is finding them. Although resources are starting to become available for survivors, it's still rare for there to be support groups and specialized counseling available for partners. Fortunately, more and more counselors, rape crisis centers (which provide some of the best services around), and religious and family service agencies are starting to look at the needs of survivors *and* their immediate families.

If you're interested in joining a support group, though, you may have to wait a long time for someone to set one up for you. Take the initiative to start one on your own. I strongly recommend this. Nothing takes the place of peer group support. To sit in a small group with ten other partners (or even over coffee and donuts with one other partner) and to talk about your frustrations, successes, failures, and strategies for dealing with your in-laws can relieve a tremendous sense of isolation and loneliness. One partner explained: "Hearing other people talk about the same thing has been great. Feeling that I'm not alone, that I'm not the first person in history to go through this, being able to call and get some perspective and validation from that other person, has been invaluable."

Many of us feel we have to bear our burdens alone or aren't used to talking about family problems, but this is a problem that needs to be talked about. You need at least one other person (aside from the survivor in your life) with whom you can honestly discuss your feelings. (See page 162 for more on choosing that person.) And if you are resourceful, you will be able to find that person, even in Duluth.

Partners' groups have formed out of one-day workshops, through ads in the newspaper, or from notices put up on the bulletin board at local counseling centers. If the survivor in your life is a member of a support group, you can ask if he or she would find out if there are any other partners who might like to get together. Once you get together, you can choose topics to discuss and meet on your own, or you can hire a facilitator who can run group meetings and provide information and resources.

There is nothing as effective as talking to someone else in your shoes. You may be in individual therapy to deal with issues from your own childhood or you might choose a round of couples' counseling with your partner. Those can both be invaluable. But the support of other partners should be your backbone. In a partners' group, you give yourself permission to whine, complain, get angry, be proud, share experiences, brag about how great you are, and help each other. This is something you can create whether you're in Dubuque, Iowa; Ketchikan, Alaska; or New York City.

Go ahead. You need it.

Sometimes I feel like she's joined this club and I'm not qualified to be a member. I feel left out and it's kind of lonely sometimes.

This feeling is a common one. If your partner is actively involved in her healing, her identity as a survivor, though painful to her, is also giving her a path through which she can reclaim her life. She has support, friends, and resources to help her in her healing. You may have very little by comparison. Her life is full of healing activities. Yours, which perhaps was once filled with her, is now relatively empty, and you haven't had any say in it. It's easy to feel lonely. Not just lonely, but downright envious at times.

Out of all the partners' workshops I've ever done, one partner stands out the most clearly. After a day of tears and laughter, bonding and problem-solving, I asked if anyone had anything else to say. A woman stood up in the back of the room and raised her hand. I nodded at her to talk. "I'm experiencing something and I haven't heard anyone else talk about it," she told the group. "Before I leave today, I want to know I'm not the only partner who feels this way." She paused. Her voice had that pre-cracking, trying-not-to-waver sound. "I'm ashamed to say this," she went on, haltingly. Everyone turned toward her, beaming support, giving her the room to speak. "Well, it's just that, well . . . I don't know how to say this, but sometimes, I feel jealous. I feel awful saying this. She's immersed in such pain and horror. She's working so hard, and I'm so proud of her. I feel terrible about what she's going through, about what was done to her. My own life was so easy by comparison. I was never abused at all. No one ever raped me or beat me or told me I was a stupid shit, and to tell you the truth . . ." Here her voice trailed off. She swallowed once, and then continued softly, tentatively, "Sometimes I wish someone had." She paused, struggling for words. "I don't really mean that, and it's hard to say what I actually do mean, but I think it comes down to the fact that she has something to pin her pain on." She stopped again. We all breathed with her in the silence. "I don't have anything to pin my pain on, and I wish I did. I feel lonely and scared, too, sometimes. I blank out and panic and feel the terrible hostility of the world crushing in on me. I don't have an excuse. I don't have a reason. I can't say it's because I'm an incest survivor or because my father beat me with a belt when he was drunk. I'm just human, and sometimes I just feel scared or lost or alone in the world. I came from a good family, and I feel bad sometimes. Incest survivors don't have a corner on feeling bad . . ." Here she paused again, looking around at the room of partners. People were nodding silently. A few had tears running down their cheeks. She drew in a ragged breath and continued, "She has a support group and books and a whole community of survivors backing her up. I don't begrudge her any of that. I'm glad she has support. But I wish I did too. She knows her enemies—and her allies. I know nothing—only that I hurt. And that's why I'm jealous. I don't wish I was abused, and I know it's terrible that it happened to her, but sometimes I still feel jealous. I feel stupid saying this, but I need to know if anyone here knows what I'm talking about."

There was a silence in the room. It went on for a long time. I broke it as gently as I could. I asked softly, "How many people here can relate to what she just said?" Hands went up all over the room. People held still, breathing together, in recognition of a truth that had been acknowledged. "Yes," I said, turning to the woman who had spoken. "Your feelings are perfectly natural, and I admire your courage in saying them out loud."

It is hard being human. All of us have pain. All of us feel anguish. All of us have days where life is a terrible struggle. This is the human condition. Sometimes survivors are under the misconception that healing will lead them to a place where they feel happy all the time, as if happiness was a permanent goal we could strive for. Or they assume they never would have felt empty and alone if they hadn't been abused. Every negative feeling in life is chalked up to sexual abuse. That's not the way it is. There is pain in life, and no amount of healing is going to take it all away. Being alive means terrible storms, brilliant sunsets, cloudy days, and sunny afternoons. There's no escaping it. It's all we have: each moment, each feeling, and the constancy of change.

We don't have to have a reason for our feelings. They just are. If you feel elated or joyous or wrapped in a deep peace, you didn't necessarily do anything in particular to deserve it. Nothing had to happen to make you feel that way. And there's nothing you can do to hold on to it. If you feel jealous or lonely or desolate, it doesn't always mean something's wrong. It may just mean that you are awake and alive and willing to live fully. That's the best any of us can do.

ALLIES IN HEALING

"You have to go into it knowing it's your problem too."

"Be ready to work. It's going to be a struggle, but that struggle can be a bonding between the two of you."

I have the feeling I've been invited to play baseball, and suddenly I don't know the rules. They've changed.

This is a very common feeling among partners. You're walking along and your life is going one way, and suddenly everything changes. The person you've loved and relied on suddenly falls into a deep hole. That hole is called "incest" or "child sexual abuse." Your partner enters a world you know nothing about. Instead of being just a regular person, she's become a "survivor." She's exploring a new identity that has nothing to do with you. Everything she's doing is new and foreign, And you don't have any say in it. Your relationship is changing. You don't understand why. Things don't fit anymore. You feel insecure and confused.

It's shocking when the person you love tells you that she was sexually abused as a child. If you haven't been exposed to abuse before, the very idea of anyone abusing a child is shocking. If you haven't thought about it in terms of your partner, you have to assimilate a whole new reality. You may have to deal with the fact that she never told you before. Maybe you love her abuser. You've played cards with him after dinner every Saturday night. Now you're supposed to accept the fact that he raped her? No wonder you feel bewildered.

The person you thought you knew the best in the world is changing radically. Her feelings, her interests, her behavior, and her responses to you are all changing. You find yourself thinking, "She's not the person I thought she was." And in a way you're right. She's discovering a part of herself that she left far behind. It's been buried for years. Yet it's as much a part of her as all the rest.

If you're in shock over these revelations and changes, you need validation. The fact is, your world has changed. You're not crazy. The bottom *has* just dropped out of your world. You didn't choose it, but your life and your relationship has changed. Things aren't ever going to be the way they were before.

If you're the kind of person who's taken pride and found security in being a strong person whose life is under control, dealing with child sexual abuse will be particularly challenging to you. There's nothing predictable about what the survivor (and by extension, you) will be dealing with for the next few years. You will be challenged to your limits; but you will also have opportunities for growth and intimacy that go beyond anything you've ever experienced.

You are absolutely right. The rules have changed. Get some support for yourself in this bewildering time.

Why me? Why do I have to sacrifice so much for something I never had a part of? I didn't abuse her. Why am I stuck with the results?

This is a very difficult question because there is no one right answer. The fact that you're with a survivor may be deeply connected to your own childhood history. Then again, it might not be.

I remember a talk by JoAnn Loulan, author of *Lesbian Sex* and *Lesbian Passion*. She was discussing the way couples meet. She said, "It's almost like we're all in a big room. Someone raises their hand and says, 'I'm an alcoholic. I'm looking for a co-alcoholic.' Another person says, 'I was physically abused as a kid. Anyone here into violence?' A third calls out, 'I'm terrified of abandonment. I'm looking for someone who can't make a commitment.' I'm not sure how we find each other," Loulan went on, "but we sure seem to find each other."

The underlying reasons we choose a particular partner are rarely clear to us when we first enter a relationship. Yet they often play a strong role in our selection of a mate. Partners who've been caretakers in their own families may be drawn to survivors who seem particularly fragile or needy, so they can fulfill a familiar role. Partners who need a lot of control may choose a survivor who seems passive and dependent. And partners who don't want to face their own pain may unconsciously choose a survivor as a way to overshadow their own problems.

On the other hand, sexual abuse may simply be one of the wild cards you've drawn in life. Your partner didn't fill out a qualifications checklist when you got involved. You fell in love with someone who was sexually abused. It may have just been the luck of the draw. So many women and men are sexually abused that I'm surprised when I meet someone who's never had an intimate relationship with a survivor.

Part of any relationship is dealing with the trials each of you goes through in life. Your trial right now is sexual abuse, but it might have been some other grief. Your partner could have become sick and died. You might have developed a debilitating disability. You might have lost a child or been unable to conceive one. There are many tragedies and challenges in life, and you don't get to choose which ones cross your path. At least with sexual abuse, you're dealing with a problem which can be, to a large part, resolved.

Remind yourself that abuse is something that happened to your partner. It is not who she is. You are not with a damaged person; you're with a good person who had something terrible happen to her. The abuse wasn't her fault. She didn't want it or choose it. She's stuck with it, and for the moment, so are you. Her job right now is to fight back against the effects of the abuse. You can choose to fight back with her. Or you can walk away. Walking away doesn't guarantee that you won't be thrown another wild card in the course of your life—you will be, inevitably.

There is no one answer to the question "Why me?" You will have to look inside yourself and come up with your own answers. Personally, I'm a realist. I am not a believer in the "everything happens to us so we can grow" school of thought. I believe in random tragedy. I don't think everything happens to us for a reason (so we can evolve spiritually, learn lessons, get enlightened). I don't think you hooked up with a survivor because you needed to on "a higher plane." These things just happen. It's life. See if you can rise to the situation with your spirit and humanity intact.

I don't know the survivor anymore because he doesn't know who he is. What can I do? How can we salvage our relationship?

Allow it to change.

Change is basic to life. Our lives are a series of transitions—from childhood to adolescence to adulthood to old age to death. Each stage has its turmoil, uncertainty, anguish, opportunities, and eventual resolution. Everyone who lives with attention and openness experiences cycles of growth and change. We all have times in our lives where we ask deep and probing questions about who we are, what we're doing, and why. Having your life torn open and reassembled periodically is part of the human condition—it's not the exclusive territory of survivors.

In order to last, every relationship has to weather these crises. This year it's the survivor's turn. Next year it may be yours. You never know when you will be wrenched out of your daily life by some event or circumstance that starts you asking, "Why?"

Of course, we'd all like to go through life's changes and transitions at the exact same rate as our partner. It would make things easier. (Or would it? Sometimes it's nice to have someone providing the stability.) But there's no guarantee that you'll be in sync with your partner. Sometimes you will be; other times you'll be with a stranger for awhile until you get to know each other all over again. Hopefully, your relationship will weather these shifts. But sometimes one of you hits a turning-point and changes in such radically different ways that it no longer works to be together. (If this is happening for you and you're thinking of leaving your relationship, see page 87.)

As much as you can, open yourself to the possibilities of change. If you're with a survivor who is actively healing from child sexual abuse, you're in a growing relationship; one in which self-awareness, feelings, and personal needs are valued. Being open to new parts of yourself can be one of the benefits of being a partner. Take advantage of the opportunity to question patterns and assumptions you've taken for granted in your own life.

Even though the survivor's changes may scare or threaten you, let her willingness to risk inspire your own journey. Don't get left behind trying to hang on to the way things were. Do some exploring and changing of your own. Then see where the two of you end up.

Why do survivors need to go to therapy and support groups all the time? It seems if one wants to get over something of this magnitude, they should just let go. It seems to me that these groups just keep reminding them of their past.

The attitude expressed in this question is held by many well-meaning people who want to be supportive but don't understand the basics of healing from child sexual abuse. Someone they love is in pain, and they want the pain to go away. They wrongly assume that the pain started when the survivor started *talking* about the abuse. It didn't. It started with the abuser and the things he or she did. The survivor has been hurting all along; it's just that he's finally identified the reason for his pain. To an outsider, it can seem like paying attention to the problem *is* the problem, but focusing on the hurt (for a time) is actually the only way to really get through it.

There's a big difference between repression and denial on one hand, and healing on the other. You can push away something that has hurt you, but it continues to fester unless you address the injury at its source. Most survivors have spent their lives trying to forget, to "let the past take care of itself," to "let bygones be bygones." Unfortunately, the effects of abuse don't go away that easily. When survivors shove the abuse away, it continues to leak out into their lives—showing up in poor self-esteem, self-destructive behavior, troubled relationships, work problems, and difficulties with sex.

If it were possible to get over the effects of sexual abuse by pretending it didn't happen or by forgetting it, most survivors would gladly sign up for a class in memory loss. Healing is not something any of us choose easily or comfortably. Going to therapy and support groups isn't fun. It's agonizing. Ellen Bass recently told me that members of one of her incest survivors' groups had renamed our book, *The Courage to Heal*, "The Carriage to Hell," because the process of healing is so incredibly painful.

It is not, however, necessary for survivors to be in support groups for the rest of their lives. The point of healing is to get through the pain, and on to other parts of life. But that process can't be rushed or hurried. It's essential that survivors get the support they need for as long as they need it. To someone on the outside, this may be hard to accept, but it's only by fully facing the pain and rage and terror that survivors become free to move on.

As a partner, you will have to come to terms with the fact that the abuse needs to be dealt with. Until you do, the two of you will be warring over something the survivor needs very much. You feel resentful and he feels unsupported. Getting locked into this kind of struggle is fruitless and hurtful to both of you.

Try not to stand on the sidelines, tapping your foot, waiting for it to be over. Get involved. See what there is for you to learn.

You need to find a source of strength, patience, and perspective that will help you through this difficult time. Spend time in nature. Notice the way things have a fallow season, a cold and lifeless time, before they can bloom again. Think about the reasons you love your partner. This is a time when faith—in the survivor's essential strength and your own determination—can help you through a lot of lonely, troubled nights.

What forms of denial exist for partners? How does this affect them and their relationships?

There is nothing inherently wrong with denial. All of us need denial to protect us from things we're not ready to face or that we can only face in small doses. If I need to take a medical test to determine whether I have a serious illness, but have to wait two weeks to get the results, I can either spend two weeks fretting and worrying or I can try to put it out of my mind until I find out there's something substantial to worry about. I call this "small *d*" denial. It's survival. It makes sense. Both partners and survivors need "small *d*" denial to make it through the day.

"Big *D*" denial is something else. It means never facing something that needs to be faced. It's "small *d*" denial frozen in place. "Big *D*" denial means never going to the hospital for the test at all. It means refusing to believe that the abuse ever happened. To be helpful as a partner, you'll need to overcome the types of "big *D*" denial described below.

On the most basic level, partners deny that the abuse occurred at all. They don't believe the survivor when she talks about her childhood experiences. They refuse to believe that it's possible—and in fact common—to forget the abuse happened and then to remember it years later. If the survivor doesn't have crystal-clear memories, partners sometimes discount or minimize the clues that are there. They assume the survivor is exaggerating or making it up. They say things like "You're just saying this to jump on the incest bandwagon." Or they think, "She's crazy." Or they don't say anything at all, their lack of belief expressed in silence. This is denial at its most basic level.

Sometimes partners take in the information superficially but don't really assimilate that anything damaging happened. They accept the facts of the abuse but minimize the trauma. They say things like "Oh, it happened so long ago," or "It was just your swimming coach and it only happened once." This is denial of the fact that the abuse mattered, that traumatic events from childhood have a real and lasting impact. They assume the survivor has a choice in dealing with the abuse, that she could just as easily "let go" and "put it behind her."

Partners also deny that the abuse has anything to do with them. They may acknowledge that the survivor has a problem, but don't see the need to get involved themselves. They don't want to look at the ways the abuse is affecting them or their relationship. Nor do they see themselves playing any role in the survivor's recovery. They don't take the time to learn about the dynamics of child sexual abuse. They resist making any accommodations or changes in their own lives. Rather, they want the survivor to "get fixed" on her own, the quicker the better.

As a form of self-protection, partners often refuse to realize how long it actually takes to heal. This usually manifests itself in their hurrying the survivor along or refusing to make the kind of shifts that are necessary when facing a long-term crisis. "Once it was identified," one partner told me, "I wanted to put it behind us and move on. I'm still waiting for her to say, 'I'm better now.'" This is a classic form of denial that keeps partners from getting involved.

Siding with the abuser or the survivor's family is a form of denial that is particularly damaging for the survivor. Partners say, "But I know so-and-so. He couldn't have possibly done that to you." Because they don't hold the offender responsible, partners sometimes refuse to change their relationship with the offender when the survivor desperately needs them to. They minimize the survivor's need to separate from her family. They don't think it will do any harm if the kids stay alone with Grandpa. This form of denial can result in real tragedy when another generation gets abused. (For more on this, see pages 214 and 224.)

Lastly, partners sometimes use the fact that their spouse was sexually abused as something to hide behind. Once sexual abuse is identified as an issue, partners sometimes blame all the couple's problems on the abuse. Instead of taking responsibility for their role in the relationship's troubles, they assume that every communication problem, sexual difficulty, or struggle over control arises from the survivor's abuse history. This is a convenient way to avoid looking at their own issues, addictions, and need to make changes. This may include denying their own childhood abuse.

If you want to be a supportive partner, breaking through your own denial will be your first task. Although it isn't easy, it is possible to move from a place of disbelief to one of supportive acceptance. Frequently, it takes time for survivors to believe their own memories;

you may need time too. If you're struggling to believe the things the survivor has told you or to accept the fact that the abuse is still affecting her, keep working at it. With support and information, you will eventually be able to believe her fully.

What if I'm willing to work through the abuse but he isn't?

If you're in a relationship with a survivor who isn't ready to actively deal with his abuse, there's not much you can do. You can encourage him, point him in the direction of resources, tell him how his stance affects you, but ultimately, the survivor is the one who has to make the decision to heal. The commitment to heal is a difficult choice, and if the survivor isn't ready to make it or doesn't think he needs to, you can't force him. In order to heal, he has to harness his will and his energy. That doesn't happen without a whole lot of determination.

People don't usually heal willingly. They don't make a commitment to heal because it's fun to grow. They do it because they're in so much pain, they're forced to. The option of not healing and staying stuck where they are becomes more painful than the pain and fear involved in healing. That's the point at which most people are motivated to heal.

If the survivor in your life hasn't reached that point, he may not be ready to deal with the abuse. He may never be. There's no guarantee that he will wake up a year or two from now, suddenly ready to look at the impact abuse has had in his life. You may be with a survivor who will continue to deny or minimize the abuse. On the other hand, he may just need more time.

If you can see that abuse is affecting your relationship and you're with someone who doesn't want to explore that possibility, there are some questions you'll need to ask yourself: "Am I willing to be intimate with someone who won't look at something which may be keeping us from getting closer? If he isn't willing to face the abuse, what does that say about the way he'll deal with other issues that arise between us? Am I getting enough from the relationship *as it is now* to stay over the long haul?"

You'll also need to take a hard look at yourself and the role you play in the relationship. There may be things that you're doing—subtle or overt—which are getting in the survivor's way. Sometimes the survivor's hesitancy has to do with a perceived (or actual) lack of safety. His reluctance to tackle the issue of sexual abuse may have to do with the fear that you'll leave if he becomes too needy or vulnerable. Ask yourself honestly, "Will I stick with him if he starts healing and becomes distracted, upset, and self-absorbed? Have I given him the message that he needs to be 'strong and together'?"

Other times survivors resist dealing with the abuse because they're being pressured. Couples sometimes get into a power struggle in which they try to control each other. Ask yourself: "Do I have a self-improvement agenda for the survivor? Do I think I know what's best for him? Do I frequently focus on what he needs to work on, instead of on problems in my own life?" If you answered yes to any of these questions, back off. Give the survivor room to examine his own life and draw his own conclusions.

One of the best places to get support for "backing off" is Al-Anon. Designed for the spouses of alcoholics and drug abusers, Al-Anon teaches its members to focus on their own needs and feelings, instead of the needs of the addicts in their lives. Even though the survivor may not have a drug or alcohol problem, Al-Anon can be a great place to develop the sense of detachment and independence you need. Instead of fixating on the survivor and his problems (or his unwillingness to deal with them), you'll be encouraged to focus on the things you need to work on in your life. That's the best and only really effective thing you can do to change your relationship.

Is it common for partners to be survivors as well but not to recognize it?

This is a scenario I've seen many times. When I was first remembering my abuse, my partner had an extremely difficult time dealing with my issues and problems as a survivor. After half a year of struggling, she left the relationship, saying she couldn't be with someone who didn't want to have sex. Several years later, when I was starting to emerge from the crisis of remembering my abuse, I found out that she was having memories of her own. It turned out that she was a survivor, too. My experience, in fact, had hit too close to home for her. This is fairly common. The partner who hasn't yet remembered feels extremely threatened, and either negates the survivor's experience or flees in terror.

Other times, the survivor's scrutiny of childhood issues leads the partner to ask questions about things he or she may have blocked out while growing up. Noah, whose story appears on page 258, explains:

> In the course of everyday living, I'm discovering things that make me reconsider my childhood. Every day I have the reminder of a survivor talking about her upbringing. I have the tendency to say, "Oh, poor you. I didn't have that." But then I have to stop and think, "Well, I'm far from perfect. I have a lot of problems. My family must not have been perfect."

The fact that one person has cleared space to look at old hurts makes room for the partner to look too. Noah adds:

> When we first got together, we used to fight a lot. She'd say, "You're doing this. You're doing that." My first instinct was, "No, it's all your fault." After a while I started to ask myself, "Why do I lie all the time?" I lie a lot. "Why do I hide so many things?"

Since one of the ways survivors remember is by hearing other people talk about abuse, one person's memories can stimulate the other's. If you find yourself extremely disturbed when the survivor talks about abuse (more than just your basic empathetic response), it may be resonating with some buried experience of your own. (See page 132 for more on this.)

If you're with a survivor, it doesn't necessarily mean that you were sexually abused or battered or have some other hidden trauma that needs to be unearthed. But it may. When you're involved with someone who's in an active healing process, it's going to affect you. You can't help but begin to ask yourself some questions about your own childhood. You may be one of the lucky people who came from a "basically good home." But be open to the possibility that the survivor's self-exploration may lead you to stumble on some buried pain of your own. The survivor may not be the only one in your relationship with healing to do. One partner put it simply:

> First I blamed her for everything. Then we blamed the abuse and her father for everything. And then we recognized that I had history, too.

If my partner and I are both survivors, how can we balance our needs?

When both members of a couple are survivors, you can either become powerful allies or terrible foes. At its best, a two-survivor relationship affords you the opportunity to relate intimately with someone who really understands, to whom you don't need to explain, who can support and make room for your healing because she knows what you're going through and where you're headed. At its worst, you get trapped in competition, comparisons, and fighting. You become tangled in your most destructive patterns and reenact the dynamics of the abuse between you. When you're partnered with a survivor, you're likely to experience both of these extremes at times, and everything in-between.

A lot depends on where each of you is in the healing process. If one of you has been working on these issues for years and is feeling fairly resolved, and one of you is just beginning, the more resolved person can offer a lot of guidance, information, and reassurance to the one who's just beginning. The hitch is that the person who's struggled to get through her sexual abuse work, who's finally in a stable place where she can focus on her present life, may not want to deal with the issues all over again. The first survivor may want a well-deserved break from dealing with sexual abuse. (See "Lorraine's Story" on page 274 for an example of this.) She may have more pressing issues to deal with in her own life or she might be trying to break a lifelong pattern of taking care of others. As a result, she may want her partner to do all the major healing work with other people.

Sometimes the first survivor will be in a place in her own life where she can afford to be more involved, more generous. She may want to get in there with her partner and roll up her sleeves. Then she'll have to deal with the question of whether her partner will let her; sometimes survivors have trouble letting their partners in on their deepest pain.

If you're both heavily in the midst of dealing with the abuse, you're going to need a lot of support. You'll need to develop some skills in negotiation, if you don't already have them, because there will be lots of times you want your partner to be there for you, or vice versa, and it won't be possible. (For help with negotiation skills, see page 169.) As much as possible, take turns being in those deep, painful places. If both of you are needy children at the same time and no one is the adult, you've got two unsupervised kids going at it, and that generally means trouble.

Don't assume that your partner's issues are the same as yours. Don't assume you know exactly how she feels or what she thinks. She may not need to heal the same way you do; her path may be very different from yours. Don't get trapped telling her what she needs to do or when she needs to do it. Although there may be similarities in your experience, you didn't grow up in the same family. You're different people. You have different strengths and weaknesses and have relied on different coping mechanisms. You're each going to have to find your own way. There is no one formula for healing from child sexual abuse.

Your first responsibility in healing is to yourself. Accept the fact that there will be times when you'll have to focus exclusively on your own healing; times when you can't offer your partner any kind of support. At times like those, you'll be more like companions traveling on parallel tracks. You'll be busy doing your work and she'll be busy doing hers, and you may not be able to do more than witness each other's changes. When you're both heavily self-absorbed and don't have much to give, you're each going to have to get your primary support somewhere else. Don't expect it from each other or you'll end up feeling disappointed, resentful, and abandoned. When you can't be there and have nothing to give, try to be a neutral observer or friend, rather than an angry obstacle.

If you reach a point where it seems like you're bringing out the worst in each other, get outside help. A couples' counselor can assist you in analyzing the ways you're trapped and in developing strategies for getting through the hard places. He or she can guide you in setting ground rules that will enable you to interact in a healthier way. (But you don't have to wait until you're in a crisis to go for couples' counseling; all couples can benefit from periodic help with communication, sex, and staying close.)

Remind yourself that there is more to life and to your relationship than healing. Make sure you have time together that is not focused on sexual abuse. Schedule time-outs, periods when you agree not to talk about it. This is mandatory for your survival as a couple. There has to be more to your union than two battered people trying to become whole. Go bowling. Take a vacation. Read mystery novels out loud. Renew an interest in something you shared while you were courting. Also, remember your sense of humor. I don't think any couple can make it through the drama of two people healing from sexual abuse if they don't find a way to laugh together.

Ultimately, loving and healing with another survivor can be a very positive experience. You're working toward a common goal, share a frame of reference, and have both made personal growth a priority. This doesn't mean, however, that your relationship will last forever: healing requires a willingness to allow change and honor individual needs; sometimes couples find themselves moving in different directions and decide to separate. That doesn't mean they failed; it means they grew together as long as they could.

Other couples come through the healing crisis feeling closer than before. Healing together can create a strong bond and give you a sense of confidence in your capacity to handle difficult problems. Knowing you've made it through the rough places can forge a powerful foundation for the years when your relationship won't revolve around sexual abuse.

What's the best way (if there is one) of getting through all this without ending up hating each other?

When one person in a couple (or both) is healing from child sexual abuse, it's easy to become polarized and to start blaming each other for the pain and frustration you're experiencing. It's crucial that you direct your anger and frustration toward the abuser and the society which allows abuse to continue, not toward each other. You need to be allies working toward a common goal (better communication, a relationship not overshadowed by sexual abuse, shared sexual intimacy). Remember that the survivor was the victim of a crime, that it is not her fault that she is having flashbacks and can't hold up her end of your relationship right now. The survivor needs to remember that you are not the enemy, not the abuser, and that you can't be expected to be a perfectly supportive partner with no needs of your own.

Paradoxically, a greater sense of independence may be one of the most important keys to staying together. The more the two of you rely solely on each other, the more stress you put on your relationship. It's crucial that you each develop outside support. You need a place (or people) you can go to when you need to express your frustrations, your doubts, your anger. The survivor needs support from a variety of other sources so you aren't the sole provider of reassurance, nurturing, information, and safety.

Accept the fact that you're making a free choice to stay in a relationship with a survivor. That way you'll feel less trapped, and therefore, less resentful. The more you see the healing process as a mutual journey in which you both have things to learn, the more patience and compassion you'll have for each other. One partner, Jack, explains:

Be prepared to confront yourself. A lot of the things you have to deal with will test you. They're probably not what you thought life and marriage were all about. The message for me has been, "Get your own house in order." For a long time, I had us polarized: the survivor was the person causing all these problems and I was the victim. When you believe that you're a victim, you can just wallow in self-pity.

You don't have to *do* anything. It was easy for me to put the survivor in the tormentor's role: "She's the one who hates sex. She's the one who flips out when you say the wrong word. I can't walk behind her." But when I started accepting responsibility for my own emotional well-being, my own identity, and my own life, I got out of that trap. We became allies, instead of enemies. [For more of Jack's story, see page 245.]

The survivor in my life is not my spouse and never has been. We are best friends. Our relationship is sisterly, nothing sexual. How can I help her?

Whether you are partners who are best friends or are "just" best friends, you play a crucial role in the survivor's life. As a best friend, there's a lot you can do to help her. Love her. Remind her that the abuse happened to her; it isn't who she is. Tell her why you think she's the best.

Don't let her withdraw or push you away just when she needs you the most. Insinuate yourself in her life. Track her down and hang in there. Be your irresistible, charming (and sometimes cranky) self.

Bring her flowers. Cook her dinner. Offer to sleep over so you can stay up, listen to music, dance, read poems out loud, cuddle, and talk about your dreams. Let her cry in your arms.

Have adventures together. Encourage her to take risks and dare more.

Call her every day, or every other day. Twice or three times on hard days. Send her postcards with silly pictures on one side and affirmations on the other.

Tell her it will be okay, that you're sure she can make it through all this.

You've developed a history with your best friend, and history enables you to be a great meter of reality. You have perspective; you can be the inside yardstick. Remind her that she's actually made progress in the last year. Document the specifics. As a best friend, your opinions are invaluable: you can tell her when she's attracted to someone who's dangerous for her, remind her of all the ways she's successfully dealt with panic before, and offer to go with her to visit her brother because you already know how difficult it will be.

Survivors who have best friends are on very good ground. A survivor can pay a therapist or join a support group (great things indeed), but her best friend is there because of loyalty and love, not because she's being paid or because she shares a particular pocket of agony. With you as a best friend, the survivor gets to learn a lot about genuine love and acceptance.

If you're not also the survivor's partner, don't belittle your relationship or your importance in her life because you're "only friends." Many survivors have maintained friendships that have been more long-lasting and influential than any of their love relationships. You're a crucial part of her support system. You play an important role in her life. (And she in yours.)

Keep your relationship current. Make sure you keep things reciprocal so you'll want to keep being best friends. Ask her for things you need, too.

Take your commitment to each other seriously. Work on problems or issues that come up between you. Best friends need tune-ups just like other relationships. But don't forget to have fun. She probably doesn't laugh with anybody the way she laughs with you. And sometimes that's the best therapy of all.

MY NEEDS AND
FEELINGS

"Don't take care of the survivor. That's not your job in life. Take care of yourself."

"What are you going to do when the survivor doesn't want to be touched? How are you going to feel when it's impossible for her to be responsible in any facet of her life?"

"If you're not careful, you can be swallowed up by the survivor's needs and pain and struggles. Separate what's happening to you from what's happening to him. Take care of yourself."

How do I explore my own needs while my home is so full of her pain and her healing?

It's not easy, but it's necessary. In fact, it's critical. When you're involved with a survivor of child sexual abuse, it's easy to focus all the energy of the relationship on the survivor's needs. Healing from child sexual abuse is dramatic, demanding, and compelling. Particularly in the beginning, you'll be faced with crisis after crisis. The survivor is dealing with memories, confronting family members, and facing the horror and pain of sexual abuse. Your own needs pale in comparison. Of course you want to be supportive. You want to be there for your partner. So you put your own feelings aside, saying, "I can wait." You let your needs slip into the background, until they go underground entirely. This is where you make your biggest mistake, both for yourself and for the relationship.

It's natural to offer practical help and encouragement to someone you love. Part of a loving friendship or partnership is a willingness to help and support your partner. There's nothing wrong with letting your partner lean on you occasionally. As long as you get to lean back. The problem arises when the giving is one-sided; when you consistently diminish yourself and your needs to serve someone else. Or when you use your "helping" as a shield from your own feelings, needs, and truths.

In reality, you are half of the relationship; you have half of the needs. Although your needs may not be as compelling, they are still important. If you consistently give and don't receive back, you are bound to end up feeling resentful and angry.

In a short-term crisis, it is appropriate to put your needs aside temporarily. When there's a death in the family, a medical emergency, or an acute illness, it's natural to step in and do what's needed without thinking of yourself. But when you're dealing with chronic illness or a crisis that extends over a period of years, a different strategy is needed. You can't live successfully in an extended state of emergency, burying your own feelings and needs whenever they emerge.

Child sexual abuse is not a short-term crisis. Although there may be periods of crisis within the healing process which require an emergency response, for the most part you are facing slow healing over a period of years. You will have to learn to balance your own needs with the demands of the situation. As a couple, you and the survivor will have to find a way to acknowledge your needs, even if they can't be met fully in the moment. Eventually, you'll learn to take turns.

This may be very threatening to the survivor. When I run groups for partners I ask everyone a series of questions in the beginning to loosen things up, to let people know that other people in the room share their experiences. Toward the end of the list, I ask, "How many people came here of their own free will? How many experienced a small degree of coercion? A large degree?" Hands go up and people laugh. It's a way to break the tension at the beginning of the day.

When I was in Minneapolis recently, a man raised his hand at the end of my list of questions to add one of his own, "How many people here wanted to come, but the survivor didn't want you to?" Several hands went up. This was a question that had never occurred to me. I wanted to know more so I asked a few of the partners who'd raised their hands, "What do you mean? Why didn't your partner want you to come?"

"She was afraid I'd become too assertive."

"He thought I'd get support for being even angrier than I am now."

"She was afraid I'd stop taking care of her so much. She said there wasn't room for both of us to have needs."

"He wants this healing stuff to be about him, not about me."

We were onto something.

Survivors do not heal from child sexual abuse in a vacuum. If she wants your love and support, the survivor has to acknowledge you as a real, breathing, living, feeling person. She can't expect you to go into the deep freeze until she's done healing. Your life is being deeply affected by her abuse and she needs to acknowledge you as a person with valid needs and feelings of your own. This doesn't mean you will get everything you want, or that the survivor will immediately be able to give you a lot more than you're getting right now, but at least you won't be invisible.

Why does the survivor expect me to have no problems and be able to handle anything when he's no superman?

This is wishful thinking on the part of the survivor. He's looking for the parents he never had. He wants a nurturing, supportive, all-giving parent and he's cast you in that role. He wants you to fulfill all the unmet needs he's still carrying from childhood. But you're his partner and his equal, not his parent. He will have to get his parenting in small doses (probably with a therapist) and eventually learn to parent himself.

When survivors first begin healing, they often lose perspective on the people around them. Instead of seeing you as a distinct person with weaknesses, strengths, and vulnerabilities of your own, the survivor is probably seeing you as the abuser (see page 95) or casting you in the role of all-powerful protector because that's who he wishes you could be. One partner described this trend:

> The survivor's expectations of what would be supportive tends toward the realm of saintliness. I've gone through some more saintly periods and some less saintly periods. I'm not as in the mood to be a saint as I was when I was younger.

You don't have to be a saint. You don't have to be the perfect partner. It may be what the survivor wants, but playing the self-sacrificing martyr isn't going to do either of you any good. You get to be human—grumpy, selfish, and generous sometimes; giving, needy, and compassionate at others. At times, you'll be self-absorbed and distracted, too.

Decide how much support you can offer freely and without resentment. Then draw lines of your own. Setting limits and clear boundaries is essential to the survival of your relationship.

Also, you don't always have to feel good about being in a relationship with a survivor who's confronting his abuse. Sometimes you'll genuinely appreciate the fact that the survivor is "growing" and "slaying the dragons from the past." Other times you'll feel resentful and long for the "good old days" of D&D: denial and dissociation. Your capacity for empathy and compassion will fluctuate depending on how deprived you're feeling on any given day. This is completely natural, but the survivor may not see it that way. Used to seeing things in black and white ("If you're not supporting me one hundred percent of the time, you're betraying me"), his attitude may well be: "Love me, love my incest." You don't have to love it. You can hate it sometimes too. "I don't like this," "This is hard," and "No," are perfectly acceptable sentences to sprinkle into your conversation.

Particularly in the early stages of healing, the survivor may respond to such statements with anger and feelings of abandonment: "You're betraying me. You're letting me down. No one's ever been there for me, and this proves it. I'll never trust anyone again." But what the survivor really needs to do is grieve for the unconditional love and nurturing he didn't get as a child. No one in an adult relationship can (or should be expected to) always be there for the other person. Remind him that you're his partner, not his parent or his therapist. Continue to be an equal, feeling human being. Be caring and responsive, but have needs of your own too. Be scared. Fall apart when things get to be too much. You don't have to always be the strong one.

Our couples' counselor told me I need to set better boundaries with my wife. What's he talking about?

A boundary describes the dividing line between one person and another: You have feelings. The survivor has feelings too. Hers are not the same as yours. You have needs. She has needs. They are not the same. You each have a distinct and differing set of problems and responsibilities.

When you develop a clear sense of your own boundaries, you see yourselves as two separate, distinct people, not as one amorphous whole. You're able to tell the difference between your needs and hers, your feelings and her feelings, your problems and her problems. When you allow each other to be different, you eliminate a lot of confusion. You have less need to control each other. There is more acceptance, more room for real closeness, more opportunity for each of you to get what you really want (since you no longer have to pretend to want the same thing).

Having a sense of boundaries allows for intimacy ("Yes, you can get close to me") and also affords a sense of protection ("This doesn't feel good; get away"). When you know where you end and someone else begins, you can say yes to things you do want, and no to things you don't want. You communicate more effectively and can better negotiate differing needs.

One of the easiest ways to demonstrate the concept of boundaries is physically. If you stand still and have a person begin walking toward you, there will be a certain point at which you want them to stop—it no longer feels comfortable; they've gotten too close. If the person keeps inching closer, your feelings of anxiety and discomfort will increase. Experiment with this. Your comfort level will vary depending on the circumstances (at home, in public, at work) and your relationship to the other person. The more intimate the relationship, the more easily you can bear closeness. There are cultural variations to physical boundaries, but all of us have them.

Children learn about boundaries by the way adults respond to their needs, feelings, and bodies. Ideally, the child's body, mind, and spirit are respected and given room to grow. When she says no, her feelings are heard and acknowledged. The child learns that she has a right to set limits. When she is sad or mad, the adults around her teach her to recognize and name her feelings; they don't try to talk her out of them, as in: "No, you're not mad. You're really happy to see Uncle Bill." She learns that her feelings are valuable; that they give her important information about her world. Her body is not touched when she doesn't want it to be touched. She learns that touch is safe and pleasurable; that her body is her own.

Many of us, however, were not raised with such care and respect. We learned a far different set of lessons: "You can't say no." "You can't trust your feelings." "We're not really interested in your ideas or your point of view." When children are sexually or physically abused, the violation is even deeper: "Your body belongs to anyone who wants it." "We own and control you." Abused children lose a sense of themselves as a distinct, separate people. They feel invaded, and they are. To survive, they detach themselves from their feelings, intuition, self-awareness, and bodies, therefore losing the means to know themselves.

As adults, few of us have a healthy sense of boundaries. We either have rigid boundaries ("No one is ever going to get close to me") or weak boundaries ("Anyone can come in and take whatever they want from me; I'll be anything anyone wants me to be"). Rigid boundaries in a family lead to distance and isolation; weak boundaries, to overdependency and sometimes, further abuse. The ideal is to develop flexible boundaries, boundaries which can vary depending on the circumstance.

In order to develop clearer, more flexible boundaries in your relationship, you will need to place a higher value on listening to yourself so you can recognize your unique feelings, wants, and needs. Here's a simple exercise that can help. It will give you an opportunity to practice talking about your needs and feelings without having to justify them or compete with your partner. Just a few minutes of doing this exercise will negate the assumption that you and your partner are (or should be) feeling the same thing.

Sit down with your partner. Take a few moments to pay attention to the thoughts, feelings, and sensations you feel inside your skin. Take turns talking about what you notice going on inside your body and mind. One of you says, "I'm feeling warm. My palms are sweating." The other mirrors back that first statement, "You're feeling hot." The first person then either accepts that statement as accurate, or corrects it to make it more in line with the original statement:

"I didn't say I was hot. I said my palms were sweating and I was feeling warm." The second person then tries again, until he gets it right: "Your palms are feeling sweaty and you're warm." Then he adds an awareness of his own: "My chest is tight. I think it's scary for me to do this exercise." The first partner paraphrases this; the second partner makes necessary corrections, and the exercise continues. After a few minutes, it becomes very clear that you are not feeling and experiencing the same thing. When you're not competing for attention, you frequently discover a genuine interest and curiosity in what your partner is experiencing.

If the survivor in your life isn't ready to explore the idea of boundaries with you, begin by yourself. Start by accepting the fact that you can't heal for the survivor; her pain is her pain. Although you can comfort her and care for her, you can't take it away. Her struggles and challenges are hers; yours are yours. Set more of a priority on your needs, even if they don't appear to be as critical. Negotiate limits with the survivor. Say no more often: "No, I don't want to talk about sexual abuse right now." "No, I'm exhausted and can't listen to your memory. Could you call someone from your support group?" Say it kindly and with compassion, but say no. If you've been super available the survivor may balk, but it's actually very helpful for her to have someone with clear boundaries to bounce up against. (See "Eric's Story" on page 265 for an example.) When you start taking responsibility for your needs and feelings, you model for the survivor that she can do the same.

Developing flexible boundaries is a trial-and-error process. Often when we begin saying no, or first become aware of our needs and feelings, we become strident, rigid, or demanding. Expect that you'll make mistakes and hurt each other from time to time. Be patient. Practice. Over time you'll learn that you can maintain a sense of who you are and still respond to someone else's needs. Keep working at it. The trouble is more than made up for by the rewards: better communication, more compassion, less competition, increased respect for your differing needs, and greater intimacy.

I'm always taking care of my partner. His needs always come first. I'm a social worker and I take care of people all day. Then I come home and take care of him. When do I get my turn?

When survivors are in the midst of an active healing process, thay have tremendous needs. The survivor feels overwhelmed, terrified, disoriented, and despondent. His pain looms larger than anything else in his life. He wants you to feel it with him; to help him through it. It's easy to get sucked into his emotional vortex, to dedicate yourself to serving his needs, yet this is a sure prescription for burnout and resentment. Still, it's hard to say no. Many of us have a hard time saying no to anyone; when we love the person, it's much harder; when their pain is so visible, it's especially difficult.

One of the things that makes it even harder for us to set limits and say no is the conditioning we received as children: many of us were taught that taking care of others was the most important thing we could do in life. Sacrificing yourself for the benefit of others is standard conditioning for women and girls. Children in alcoholic homes, or in homes with parents who are ill, absorb this lesson too. If you hadn't stepped in and taken care of things as a child, your family might not have survived. You did what you needed to do, but often at a high cost to you. You squelched your own needs and feelings in order to better serve others. As one partner said:

> I have a conflict between being in a relationship and being
> my own person. It's as if I can't have one without giving
> up the other. I tend to give up things I want to do because
> the relationship demands it. I learned that as a child.

You may also be modeling yourself after a parent who played the caretaker role. One woman said, "I definitely have a tendency to give all. My mother taught me, 'If you're good and you give all, that's love.'"

When you were growing up, caretaking may have provided you with some tangible rewards. It may have ensured your own survival or given you a small measure of control over a chaotic situation. You felt valued and powerful. What you did mattered. You were needed.

CARETAKING

As an adult, you may be continuing a pattern of caretaking for similar reasons. Taking care of others may feel familiar or safe ("If I take care of others, they'll need me, and therefore, they won't leave"). It may give you an opportunity to feel good about yourself or a sense of control over your life. Yet you are also paying a price. Excessive caretaking may be one of the reasons your own needs are being neglected today.

Make a list of the positives and negatives you experience when you take care of other people. Positives might be things like: "Other people say I'm caring." "I feel like a good person." "No one gets angry at me." "Jan stays with me." Negatives might include: "I stuff my own feelings." "I get secretly resentful because my needs are ignored." "I have to do everything. It's exhausting." "I don't take enough risks. I don't challenge myself to grow."

Sometimes the fact that your needs aren't being met has as much to do with your own patterns as it does with the real and often overwhelming needs of the survivor. Recognizing the ways you've used caretaking to protect yourself, achieve control, or hide from painful realities, can help you understand your part in creating the compromising position you're in.

Gradually you'll need to reduce the amount of time you spend taking care of the survivor and increase the amount of time you spend learning about your own feelings and needs. The exercises on pages 75 and 169 can be a helpful place to begin.

How can I stop being a nice guy and make sure my own needs are met?

The first step in getting your needs met is identifying what they are. Before you do that, you have to recognize that you have needs. Some of you already know this. You're sick of waiting on the sidelines and are reading this book to figure out how to get your needs met. But if you've buried your needs for years, never learned to acknowledge them, or have shaped your life on a model of self-sufficiency, you will have to begin with the basic awareness: "I am a person. I hurt. I feel. I need."

Think about some of the most basic things you share with the rest of the human race: the need for companionship, affection, love, belonging, a sense of meaning in life. Or start by making a list of needs that spring out of your daily life: "I want help with childcare." "I want someone to talk to about what's happening in my relationship." "I want to laugh more."

Include any wants and needs you have that are currently not being met, or are not being met to your satisfaction. Include things that are practical ("I want help buying a couch"), ordinary ("I want someone to share the ups and downs of parenting with me"), personal ("I want support in planning a career change"), social ("I want someone outside my relationship I can confide in"), intimate ("I want to feel desired sexually"), and spiritual ("I want more faith that things can get better"). Include small things and large things; things that seem impossible and those that seem within your grasp. Make your list as complete as you can.

Instead of listing a specific person in connection with your want ("I want Kate to be more interested in my work"), list the need without a person attached ("I want someone to care about the details of my work"). The examples below will get you started. Copy down any that apply to you. Add any others you can think of.

- I want someone to help me solve my problems.
- I want to have more fun.
- I want to go out in nature more.
- I want time off when I don't have to be so careful about everything.

- I want to talk about how hard life is with a survivor.
- I want to make love.
- I want to feel sexy.
- I want affection.
- I want help supporting the family financially.

It is unrealistic to think that any one person is going to meet all of your needs and wants. That's why we're social creatures; why we have families, live in communities, and make friends. However, we live in a society where romantic love is idealized: if we search long enough, we will find "the one," the soulmate who is perfect for us, who will grow and change at the exact same rate we do, who loves us exactly as we are and never expects us to change, who always wants us sexually, never has bad breath or gets grouchy, and is perfectly desirable in every way. We expect our partner to fully meet us on an intellectual, physical, sexual, and spiritual basis; to be our lover, best friend, a companion, confidante, confessor, therapist, and family, all rolled into one. This sets up monumental expectations which all of us invariably fall short of. Even if your partner wasn't a survivor, these expectations would still be unrealistic. Yet many of us feel unfulfilled, unhappy, or angry if our partners don't meet all of our needs. Few of us have developed support systems which allow us to get our needs met by a variety of people.

You need help studying for an exam in a training course. You want the survivor to coach you, but she's busy at a survivors' group. Why not call a schoolmate and meet at the library? You want to go hiking. If the survivor doesn't want to, why not invite your friend Bill? Even though you might prefer to have all your needs met by the survivor, many of them can be met by other people (including yourself). Why not diversify a little? It's a sure way to get more of your needs met.

Go back through your list of needs and wants. Rate them according to the following system: Anything that involves your partner but could potentially be met by another person as well, mark with a *P*. If you can meet your own need, write down an *S* for self. If you have a need that can be met by someone other than yourself or the survivor, write *O* for other. If the needs can *only* be met by your partner, write *PO* for partner only. (Although there are probably some things only your partner can do, there are probably more that can be done by someone else as well.) Anything not marked *PO* can have more than one letter next to it:

O,P • I need to talk about how hard life with a survivor is right now.
PO • I need to make love.
S,O,P • I need to feel sexy.
O,P • I need affection.

Look over your answers. Ask yourself: "Are my expectations of the survivor realistic? What would have to change for me to meet more of my own needs? To get more of my needs met by others?" If you want to get more of your needs met, diversifying is an important way to begin. (For guidance in sharing your list with the survivor, see "Learning to Negotiate" on page 169.)

I keep feeling guilty. Why do I feel like an abuser when I state my needs?

You probably feel that way because the survivor is telling you that, either directly or indirectly. Any expression of your needs may seem abusive to her. If that's what she believes, she's wrong. Just because her abuser's needs were intrusive and abusive doesn't mean that everyone else's needs are selfish and hurtful. If she wants to be in a relationship with you, she's going to have to make room for you to have needs. (Sexuality and physical contact are special cases: if you're having this problem specifically around sex, see page 176.)

You also have to ask yourself, "Have I felt this way before? Is this a pattern I'm bringing into the relationship? Was I taught as a child that my needs were unimportant or 'too much'? Am I asking for things that are realistic?"

Bear in mind that there's a difference between stating a need and making a demand. It's unrealistic to expect that all our needs will be fulfilled on schedule, in the manner we think is best. No one has an obligation to meet our needs; they may choose to do so out of love or caring, but they aren't obliged to. If you consistently feel like an abuser, check in with yourself: "Am I sharing my simple need or making a demand? Is there any kind of threat, direct or implied, in my tone of voice or in the way I ask?" Few of us have had a lot of experience asking for what we need. We all could use some practice learning to ask gracefully. Sometimes our style of asking can have a lot to do with the way our words are received. (For help communicating effectively, see page 169.)

I have a hard time asking for support from my partner. I don't expect her to be able to ever take care of my needs because hers seem so enormous. Then I find myself getting incredibly angry at her and her family. How can I work to break this cycle?

Start asking for things you need. (If you don't know how to begin, see pages 75 and 169 for ideas.)

Also, express your anger. Vocalizing anger is a clear way to establish limits and boundaries. "I'm mad about this. It's not acceptable to me. This is how I feel!" The survivor may not be able to bear the full brunt of your rage (no one should have to, except maybe your therapist), but she needs to know that you're frustrated and angry. Find a safe place to express your deepest fury, like in a partners' group, on the handball court, or in an anger-release exercise in your counselor's office. Then go back to the survivor and tell her you're mad.

One woman described the way her healthy expression of anger clears the air in her relationship:

> When I say I'm angry at how little I get, at how hard it is,
> the survivor is relieved to know the truth, even when it's
> hard for her to hear. The more honest I am, the less she
> can believe her projections on me.

The more real you are with the survivor, the less she'll confuse you with the abuser and see you as "bad."

Anger can be an empowering force or a destructive one. Being mad doesn't necessarily lead to violence, although many people raised in violent homes believe it is. If anger is scary or threatening for either you or the survivor, you may need professional help learning to safely express anger in your relationship. (For more on the appropriate expression of anger, see page 99).

How can I share the joy I feel without ignoring the survivor's pain? How can I live my joys and sorrows without making him feel guilty and depressed?

Your personal experience of joy or pleasure or contentment—or any other feeling—need not be dependent on the survivor's pain or misery. You are each experiencing feelings. Yours may be very different than the survivor's right now. That you feel joy doesn't mean you're being disrespectful. It means you are separate human beings having different life experiences right now.

You are not responsible for what the survivor feels. You can't make anyone feel guilty or depressed. His feelings are his and yours are yours. You don't have to be in constant mourning because the survivor is. His feelings are not a barometer you have to live by. Your joy can be a reminder to him that positive feelings are possible. What good could it possibly do for you to join him in his despair?

It's possible to be aware or sensitive to the survivor's feelings and needs without feeling them with him. One woman explained, "When I have a great day, I can still feel good even if he's depressed." If you feel happy, enjoy it, because happiness doesn't last forever. The nature of feelings is that they change. Go with the shifts in your own emotional rhythm.

At the same time, be sensitive. When I'm really depressed, I find it hard to be around someone who's bubbling over with joy. But sensitivity is different than merging. Togetherness doesn't mean going through each crisis with the same feelings and at the same speed. It means respecting the feelings the survivor has, and responding to them as caring, concerned person. It doesn't mean abandoning your own experience along the way.

I'm puzzled by my own reactions when she talks about her abuse. It's almost like it's my pain, not hers.

It's natural to have a feeling, empathetic reaction when someone you love shares painful experiences and emotions with you. However, if you are consistently overreacting to the survivor's words or have an eerie feeling that they're too close to home, there may be several things going on. One is that you're over-involved in her emotional life; the boundaries between the two of you have become blurry or nonexistent. You don't see or know yourself as separate from her. You've stopped being two distinct people; you're more like two halves of a wounded whole. When you find yourself thinking, "I don't know where she stops and I begin," it means your feelings, ideas, and sensibilities have merged.

The second possibility is that you were abused yourself, and that her experience is unleashing memories and feelings connected to your own childhood pain. You may be feeling emotions that stem from an experience you haven't yet remembered or named as abuse. If you consistently feel triggered by hearing about the survivor's abuse, consider the possibility that it may have to do with something that happened in your own life. Try to foster an attitude of willingness. Say to yourself, "If there's something here to uncover, I want to know what it is." (For more, see "Partners Have History, Too" on page 56.)

I'm kind of ashamed to say so, but the topic of sexual abuse is sexually stimulating to me sometimes.

It's brave to acknowledge that reading or hearing about incest and sexual abuse sexually arouses you. This is actually a common experience, yet few people openly admit it. It's natural to be ashamed of these feelings, but acknowledging the experience is the first step in alleviating your shame.

There are several possible reasons for your arousal. The first is the way sexual exploitation is eroticized in our culture. Sex is continually linked with violence, conquest, humiliation, and pain. We see it on book and record jackets, music videos, television, magazine covers, and in our daily newspapers. Sex, and kinky sex in particular, sells. Children in erotic poses, with adult clothes, and seductive faces, sell. We've all been bombarded with these images, and they affect us. It's hard to grow up in this culture and not find violence and degradation a turn-on. The arousal you feel when you hear about sexual abuse may just be a response to the cultural exploitation of sex (and children) we've all grown accustomed to.

The second reason for your arousal may have to do with abuse you experienced as a child. Survivors are often sexually aroused when they tell their story, read about abuse, or fantasize with abuse-laden images. It's not that they like being abused; it's that the sense of arousal was imprinted along with feelings of pain, humiliation, shame, and terror. (For more on this linkage, see page 203.) Although survivors usually feel ashamed of the connection between arousal and abusive images, the associations are there, at least initially. If you find yourself aroused by stories of abuse, your reaction may point to memories of abuse stored in your own body.

The third thing to look at when considering this question of arousal is the fact that pedophiles are sexually attracted to children. They are sexually aroused by children (their bodies, their vulnerability, their innocence) and then act out that arousal, causing profound anguish for the child. Most parents who are honest will tell you that they have sensual feelings toward their children at times, but that's different than actually wanting to have sex with a child. If stories of incest and sexual abuse turn you on *and* you have any sense you might want to act on those feelings, get professional help. If you've acted out sexually with children, *stop,* and get help. If you haven't ever sexually abused a child, but you think you might, get help. You're trying to be part of the solution; don't add to the problem.

Is it possible to go one day without dealing with the survivor's issues?

Yes. If you need time off, take it. If the survivor can't stop talking about sexual abuse and you've hit your limit, spend time apart. If you're feeling inundated and overwhelmed, go visit a friend for an evening. Sleep over at your sister's house. Spend some time with people who promise not to talk about sexual abuse. Limit your conversation to recent movies, good books, and gossip from *People* magazine. Relish your escape.

Spending time away doesn't mean you're abandoning the survivor. You're doing what you have to so you can be there another day. Love doesn't mean being available to your partner twenty-four hours a day, every day. It means respecting your own needs enough so that you don't burn out.

The survivor, however, might not see it that way. He may feel utterly abandoned when you say you need time to yourself. He has a right to those feelings, although most of them have to do with childhood memories, not with you. Acknowledge his feelings, have compassion for him, but don't cave in to his need. Although it may be the hardest time for you to say no and take care of yourself, you still need to. If you don't you'll feel trapped, and ultimately may leave the relationship as your only avenue of escape.

In a genuine emergency, however, you may need to allow the survivor's needs to supercede your own. If his life and safety are in jeopardy (my definition of an emergency—you may want to come up with your own), you can't just walk out the door, saying "I need space now." You have to weigh your need for time away with the survivor's level of crisis and desperation.

Therapist Shauna Smith of Sacramento suggests using the following system of negotiating conflicting needs:

> Set up a system for negotiating ahead of time, together. One useful technique is for each of you to place the importance of a particular item on a scale of one to ten, one being "not very important" and ten being "emergency." The survivor, for example, might rate his anxiety a five, and the partner might rate his feeling overwhelmed an

eight. In this situation, the survivor could get help from his support system and the partner would take a break. If the survivor felt closer to terror, he would have indicated a nine or a ten, and then the partner would have stayed home. This is a useful technique, because each person becomes clearer in knowing and communicating the intensity of his feelings. The numbers need not be set in stone, because feelings can sometimes change from moment to moment.

This kind of scale can be a helpful guide in differentiating between genuine emergencies and uncomfortable, painful feelings. Learning to tell the difference can be an important step for the survivor (and for you) in developing a greater sense of emotional independence.

It's important, however, that the one-to-ten scale not be used as ammunition in a fight: "You're feeling a ten! Well, I'm feeling a ten, too!" Also, you may run into trouble if one of you is constantly at a high level of crisis. In that circumstance, that person's numbers might always come out higher. That's not okay, no matter how bad things are. Sometimes the person in less crisis needs to get away, regardless.

If you need to leave a situation which is bordering on an emergency, enlist some help from someone in the survivor's support system before you leave. If you can, help the survivor come up with a plan for staying safe. Then leave, letting him know where you're going and when you'll be back.

Anyone working a demanding job deserves a vacation. You do too. Find a way to get the time and space you need. It's crucial for both of you.

How do I hold on when it appears there is nothing to hold on to?

You just do. You breathe. You put one foot in front of the other. You breathe again. You reach inside yourself for strength you didn't know you had. You tell yourself, "One day, one hour, one minute at a time."

When the bottoms drops out of your world, sometimes you just have to stop and sit with it. Say to yourself: "This is my life. I'm in terrible pain. I feel lost. I don't know what to do. This is true for me right now." Keep breathing and remind yourself, "This too shall pass."

I believe the human spirit is very big. I think we are capable of a lot more than we think we are. You're being pushed to your limits right now. If you have a belief, a love, or a passion that connects you to a power beyond yourself—whether it's music, God, or the maple trees outside your window—call on that power now. Pray. Ask for help.

When the world you've known is shattered in pieces around you, do something small and concrete and manageable. Buy a chicken, put some spices on it, and put it in the oven. Wash the dishes. Clean your whitewalls. Refinish a chair, something that's completed and beautiful and steady when you're done. Keep breathing. Watch the moment pass.

Reach out to other people. You need friends right now, witnesses who can say, "Yes, it really is this bad. You're not making it up. Your life is really awful right now."

Ultimately, there's only so much other people can do. When we're in our deepest pain and despair, no one can take it away. These are your feelings of helplessness, loneliness, and confusion. I can say I understand them, but they are your feelings to feel. Sit with them. Follow them. Sometimes if we go deep enough into our pain, it changes into something else.

How do you know when to throw in the towel? What do I do about the terrible guilt I feel about leaving the relationship and thus cutting of my support of the survivor?

This is a question that many of us would rather not face, but it's a very real question of many partners. Being intimately involved with a survivor can severely test your limits. You may feel left out, frustrated, worn down. You want to be supportive, but find that you are sacrificing too much. Your needs are being ignored and you feel like you're losing yourself. There are only so many crises you can handle, so many times you can tolerate being pushed away. When your needs aren't being met, it's natural to question the relationship and to consider leaving. One man explained: "I've gotten worn down. I don't see a lot of change. She does. Things that are positive to her, like being more in touch with her anger, have negative ramifications for me." Another partner added: "I wouldn't wish this on anybody. It's not worth it." A third, a woman who left a relationship with a survivor, exclaimed, "I just couldn't keep giving unconditionally and not getting anything back."

Partners who've had a history of taking care of others sometimes question their commitment to the survivor as they get healthier themselves, wondering whether it's good for them to be in a relationship where they do so much more of the giving. Other times, both partners are so locked into unhealthy, destructive patterns that the only way out they see is to leave. One partner explained:

> My own anger, my own hurt, is so present it's hard to be
> supportive. We've built up so much history with all these
> problems, so many negative patterns have developed. Now
> it only takes a glance or slight touch for both of us to get
> our defenses all set up.

If you are thinking about leaving your relationship, it doesn't necessarily mean you are selfish or unreliable. You are hurting and in pain, struggling to deal with incredibly difficult circumstances. Give yourself room to ask the question: "Should I go or should I stay?" If you continually suppress thoughts and feelings about leaving, you'll end up feeling trapped, powerless, and resentful. Knowing that you have alternatives will give you a needed sense of control over your life. Ask yourself: "How long can I continue like this? What price will I pay if I continue to sacrifice myself? Is there room for me to grow here, too? What about my needs?" Even if you're certain you're going to stay in your relationship, asking these questions will help you become more assertive in getting your needs met.

The decision to continue or end a relationship depends on a variety of factors; your choice to stay or go will depend on a lot more than the role of child sexual abuse in your relationship. Newer relationships, those with less history or less of a shared vision, are more likely to give way under the pressure of dealing with child sexual abuse. Those with deeper roots, a stronger sense of commitment, more shared responsibilities, and a history of making it through tough times, are more likely to survive. If your relationship was rocky to begin with, sexual abuse can be the stressor that tips the balance toward splitting up.

Ask yourself the following questions: "How new is our relationship? Do we have a mutual dream? A sense of where we're going, what we want, a commitment to something bigger than our individual struggles? Are we both committed to the idea of healing and growth? What commitments or responsibilities do we share? Were we feeling confident about our commitment to each other before all of this started?" Your answers to these questions will form a base for the difficult decision ahead of you.

Not all relationships can stand the stress of one or both partners dealing with child sexual abuse. When I first had my memories, I was in a new relationship. My partner, a woman I loved very much, struggled with me through the first six months of my healing, and then broke up with me. She said she couldn't be in a relationship without sex, where her deepest needs were not being met.

When she walked out of our relationship, I was devastated. I was certain I was damaged and that no one would ever love me again. I couldn't believe she had walked out when I was the most needy and vulnerable. That was when I "hit bottom." I was having flashbacks all the time, my family accused me of lying about my grandfather, I couldn't concentrate at work, and the person I loved the most found me too damaged to be with.

When I think back to that time now, I realize my partner had to leave. It was her best option at the time. Of course, I wish she'd stayed, but the fact is I used her leaving to go deeper. I no longer had to try to "keep it together" for the sake of our relationship. I no longer had to try to be sexual (which I was failing at on a regular basis) or pretend to be interested in her needs and feelings. I wasn't capable of doing those things, and once she left, I could fall apart in peace. I mean that. I was in a terrible crisis, it's true, but there was no longer anything stopping me from going deeply into the wrenching inner work that lay before me. I was no longer distracted by needs I couldn't possibly fulfill. In the months following our breakup, I made tremendous progress.

I wish, of course, that I'd had a partner to support me through those first agonizing years. I wanted someone to hold me and love me without having any expectations that I would give anything in return. It wasn't realistic; but I wanted it desperately: to be protected and loved in a special way, for who I was and not for what I could give back. I didn't have that, but with the support of my therapist, friends, and other survivors, I found my way. And I learned something true about life in the process—each of us really is alone. Not alone in the way I was as a child spread-eagled on the bed, the alone where no one knew and no one cared. I was alone in a different way. My lover hadn't saved me. My friends couldn't save me. My therapist couldn't save me. It was my life and my pain. I had to move through it. No one else could do it for me.

As a child, the survivor already went through the worst. She survived the abuse, and the chances are, she will survive if you decide to leave. Your leaving will probably not be the thing that makes or breaks her life. I don't mean to minimize the impact your leaving might have. She would feel devastated and hurt deeply. It would bring up memories of other times she felt abandoned. She might turn on you and blame you for her pain, but the fact is, it is her pain to deal with. You couldn't heal for her while you were together. You can't while you're apart. The real core work is hers to do.

The decision to stay or go is a very big decision and a terrible choice to face. But it's better to be honest with yourself (and the survivor) than to fake a commitment that isn't there. Survivors grew up in families where they were lied to. Give the survivor the benefit of the truth. If you're thinking of leaving, talk about it. And if you ultimately do decide to leave, claim the decision as your own, based on your needs, your feelings, and your limitations. Don't blame the survivor or tell her it's her fault. Leave her with your love, your support, and her dignity intact. Then if you walk away, you can do it knowing you did your best.

DEALING WITH

CRISIS

"It just pervades everything."

"When I'm not home, I call her every hour just to see how things are going. I've thought of getting a beeper. A lot can happen in an hour."

"She always had to know where her therapist was. For two years, she always knew how and where to reach her therapist. It was devastating for her when the therapist went on vacation for a week. You thought crisis was going on before? When her therapist left, *that* was crisis."

How do I get the survivor to understand that not all frustrations, problems, or challenges have to be faced like a life-or-death struggle? Why does every stress that comes up each day seem so devastating?

When we're emotionally upset or under pressure, our ability to cope with day-to-day problems is drastically reduced. We've all had this experience. You have a sick child at home, you don't get enough sleep, your boss is upset with you, you have a fight with your spouse. You start home from work. Someone cuts you off in traffic. You start screaming and cursing and want to kill. Being cut off in traffic isn't worthy of murder, but because you're pushed to your limits, you're sure the guy in front of you deserves an instant, colorful death.

When survivors are engaged in an active healing process, particularly during periods of crisis, their ability to cope with life falters. I went through a few days like this just last week. Something happened in my family which stimulated old memories of times I felt powerless and alone. I spent several days feeling like a lost little child. I couldn't remember why I'd liked myself the week before, who I was, or what I was doing with my life. Each morning, I'd walk into my office, look around, and say to myself, "This is an office for grown-ups. I don't thing I belong here today." Then I'd go to bed and cry. Each little thing that came up became an overwhelming obstacle. A friend cancelled our vacation plans. I felt miserable and abandoned. I got in a fight with my doctor because she was late for our appointment. My best friend loaned out a book I had given her and I was furious. How could she betray me like that? These were all small things (as life problems go), but I was stretched too thin and couldn't cope with any of them. I was reacting like a six-year-old, not like a flexible, competent adult. It took a while to straighten things out when I came back to myself again. Experiencing this seven years into my healing was humbling. I'd forgotten what it felt like to fall into a hole like that. It had been over a year since I'd had that experience and I thought I was done losing the present so entirely. But even as I was humbled, I also realized how far I'd come. I spent the first couple of years I was healing feeling constantly small and vulnerable and unable to cope with daily life. Now, "falling in a hole" was clearly the exception.

When survivors are bombarded with memories and painful feelings, and are engaged in an inner struggle to heal, they often lose the capacity (at least temporarily) to respond to situations appropriately. Their emotional reactions are often overblown because the line between present hurts and old injuries disappears. They lose their sense of perspective and patience. It's like an old Plymouth with worn-out shock absorbers: every minor bump in the road sends everyone in the car bouncing up and down. One partner explained:

> As his awareness of the abuse increases, the impact on us increases too. The period we've just come through was one in which he'd be set off very quickly. Everything was a trigger.

The survivor may also be someone who thrives on crises. Many survivors grew up in families where Dad was drunk, Mom was covered with bruises, the electricity was turned off, and the baby was crying because he hadn't been fed. Danger was everywhere, and the survivor was the one person in the family who kept the whole disaster from falling apart.

The experience of life as crisis is difficult to give up. In a crisis, your adrenaline is pumping, there's a high level of excitement, and you don't have time to feel. You act on automatic. You just respond. Handling crises well can be a way to feel good about yourself. Allowing things to be quiet and responses to be appropriate means giving up a certain high that comes with drama. "If it isn't intense, I'm not really alive," is the credo for many survivors.

As a partner, this can be very difficult to deal with. You don't want every minor irritation to be a major crisis; there are enough real crises to deal with. Unfortunately, there's no easy remedy for this situation. The survivor already has his hands full; he may not be able to cope well with daily life for awhile. Part of healing is discarding outdated coping skills and replacing them with new ones that work better, but in the process there can be some shaky, vulnerable times.

There are a few things you can do. Acknowledge the survivor's feelings. Listen to him. Provide him with a reality check: "Bob cancelling your tennis game isn't the same as your father walking out on you." Share your point of view: "I don't think all this rage you're feeling really has to do with Pauline; I think a lot of it is anger at your mother for what she did to you." If the survivor is angry at you, however, you'll have to take a different approach; he won't be very receptive when you say, "This doesn't have to do with me. It's about your mother." (See page 95 for an alternative approach.)

Set an example that life doesn't have to be lived as a continual crisis. Your generally calm way of handling things may not rub off on the survivor, but it will let him know there are alternatives. But be honest about your own imperfections: if you're always calm and steady, it may mean you're shutting down your own feelings. (This is a very common response to being around someone who's continually upset.)

You also may have to just accept that you will be doing more than your share in dealing with problems for awhile. As the survivor resolves more of the pain from the past, he will be better equipped to deal appropriately with issues in the present.

Why does doing nothing seem the only safe thing to do? It seems that anything I do is almost always the wrong thing. I feel like she's always confusing me with her father.

Partners often feel as if nothing they do helps; whatever they do seems to only make things worse. If you're involved with a survivor whose memories and painful feelings are close to the surface, everything may be triggering upset, flashbacks, and rage. One partner explained:

> Since she began therapy and joined the support group, her anger is very close to the surface, and a lot of it is misdirected at me. Anything that comes close to reminding her of her father is very explosive. I'm ducking her anger a lot.

When you're in this situation, the survivor is having trouble differentiating the past from the present and everything is merging together. This can be very tough on you as a partner. There's only so long you can tiptoe around, trying to be careful. You're bound to end up feeling resentful and angry: you're sick of walking on eggshells.

Fortunately, this is a stage. It doesn't last forever.

Being with someone who is easily triggered is like being with someone who has environmental illness and is allergic to most household products. You have to go through a meticulous process of identifying each toxic substance and eliminating it from your home: scented soaps, perfumes, synthetic clothes, and detergent. It's time-consuming, but you do it. And once you do, the allergic reactions lessen.

It's similar with survivors. You locate the triggers and minimize them as much as possible. But it's a lot harder than getting rid of hairspray and deodorant: you can't erase your feelings, the inevitable conflicts that arise in daily life, the way you turn over in your sleep, your need to exist in your own house. When the survivor is going through a period of being easily triggered, your life may seem like this: You're five minutes late and suddenly you're the survivor's mother who stayed out all night drinking and rarely kept her promises to go to the park, watch the school play, or tuck her daughter in. You break a teacup and find yourself barraged with rage that rightfully belongs to the survivor's stepfather, the man who tortured her pets when she was eight. The survivor gets upset about something legitimate, and then plugs into all the times in her life anyone ever hurt her.

Therapists call this transference. You come to represent more than just yourself. The line between the past and present blurs, and the survivor can't differentiate between you and someone from the past. The triggers can be anything: you have a beard and the survivor's uncle had a beard. You are a woman with large breasts and the survivor's mother, who sexually abused her, was a large-busted woman. You raise your voice when you're angry and yelling triggers memories of her father screaming at her that she was stupid and worthless. At these moments the survivor forgets who you are and mixes you up with the abuser. You're trying to be attentive and considerate, and everything you say is being misconstrued and misinterpreted. Other times she literally sees the abuser (this is a kind of flashback; it's like you're not there anymore) or regresses and starts acting like a child: she backs up into the corner, curls her shoulders in to protect her body, as if she expects you to hit her. You feel bewildered: hitting her is the farthest thing from your mind. (For more on regression, see page 102.)

There are several things you can do if you're being confused with the abuser. Most importantly, maintain a strong presence in the relationship. If you're angry, express your anger. If you're feeling frustrated, say so. If you're feeling joyful, express your joy. If you need to set a limit, do so. Establishing limits and boundaries lets the survivor know who you are. Being a person with clearly delineated feelings, opinions, needs, and limits sets you apart from the abuser. (See "Eric's Story" on page 265 for an example of this.)

Whenever you're confused with the abuser, call for a time-out. Don't escalate. Remind the survivor who you are. Say, "Right now, I know you think I hate you, but I don't. I'm mad at you, but I don't hate you. I'm Bob. I care about you. We were having an argument and you got scared." Help talk her down.

Once the survivor "comes back," try to identify the trigger: the room was too dark; you approached her too suddenly; you came to bed smelling of beer; you made a threatening gesture in the middle of a fight. When you identify the triggers, you can often take steps to eliminate them: you can change your haircut, stop hugging the survivor from behind, quit drinking before bed, or shift your use of certain words: "I love you" might throw the survivor into a panic, reminding her of times her mother said, "I love you, honey," and then abused her. The next time you want to whisper an endearment, try "I really care about you" instead. Come up with a plan for dealing with similar triggers the next time. (Do this *before* it happens again.)

Sometimes, however, there is more to this issue than defusing triggers from the past. There may be a grain of truth in the survivor's perception of you; sometimes the survivor is reminded of the abuser because there are ways you are like him: the comparison is apt. The abuser was irrational and his anger was out of control; you haven't learned to manage your own feelings of rage. The abuser kept the survivor in a dependent position by giving and then withdrawing love; you do too. He sulked if she refused sex, and you do the same.

All of us choose partners who mirror the best and worst of our primary caregivers.[1] For survivors, unfortunately, these characteristics are often weighted toward the negative. Before you discount the survivor's accusations entirely, honestly assess the dynamics in your relationship. Ask yourself: "How do I ask for things I want? Do I make demands? Do I humiliate or badger the survivor? Do I express my anger in a threatening way? Have I ever been violent or threatened violence?"

This is one place where the survivor's sensitivity can serve your own need for healing. If you've been repeating hurtful patterns you learned as a child, you now have the chance to explore and change those patterns. This will clearly benefit both of you.

When one person in a relationship (or both) feels there are harmful or abusive dynamics going on, it's essential that you get outside help to look at them.[2] When you're caught in a struggle over power and control, it's difficult to see things clearly. You may be

---

[1] For an in-depth analysis of this important idea, read *Getting the Love You Want* by Harville Hendrix. See the bibliography for details.

[2] If there is violence going on in your relationship, the violent person needs to be stopped and the person who is being abused needs protection. Violent behavior is unacceptable and is not something to be negotiated in couples' counseling. Although most problems in relationships are caused by both people's behavior, violence is an exception.

power and control, it's difficult to see things clearly. You may be playing out the roles of victim and perpetrator and be unaware of the dynamics between you. Get some help so you can turn things around.

How do I get the survivor to understand that his constant rage and anger can only keep me at a distance?

Tell the survivor. Let him know your honest response to his anger: "I'm feeling alienated and far away." "You're scaring me right now. I can't be with you." Set limits: "I won't stay here if you keep talking to me that way. You're going to have to find another outlet for your anger."

It's appropriate (and necessary) for survivors to feel angry about the abuse, but it's also important that they learn to direct that anger at the right people. When survivors don't have safe, effective places to express their anger, it splashes all over the place, including all over you. There's a difference between respecting a survivor's healthy need for anger and letting that survivor control or abuse you with it. Constant anger can be a way to shut you out. Of course you want to protect yourself from it. Why would you want to be close to someone who's enraged all the time?

It's important to set clear boundaries where anger is concerned. It doesn't matter how healing it is for the survivor, if it's damaging to you, it's not okay. If you deserve any of the survivor's anger, deal with that part, but don't feel you need to bear the brunt of his rage. Just because he's angry doesn't mean he can express his rage wherever and however he wants.

Many survivors, particularly men, are allowed and encouraged to express only one emotion: anger. It's important that these survivors learn to feel and express sadness, grief, and vulnerability, too. One of their tasks in healing is to diversify their emotional repertoire. This means learning about new emotions and backing off of anger as the only way of expressing strong feelings. Your limit-setting and clarity about how the survivor's anger is affecting you will help the survivor attain this goal.

Although we typically think of men's rage toward women when we consider the problem of violent or uncontrolled anger in relationships, it's essential that we recognize that women are also capable of expressing anger abusively. There is battering, emotional terrorism, and violence in lesbian and gay relationships, too. If you're struggling with issues of violence or abuse in a lesbian or gay relationship, you will have fewer resources to turn to, but it's essential that you get help so you can stop the abusive anger. See page 304 for a listing of books that can help you end the violence.

What do you do when the survivor continually says, "I see no progress. I will never be a whole person." He is becoming more and more depressed.

Periods of hopelessness are natural when someone is dealing with child sexual abuse. Although things frequently feel hopeless, they aren't. Change is slow, but it does happen. The pain does not stay constant; the injuries, for the most part, are not permanent.

Sometimes feelings of hopelessness are less attached to what's happening in the present and more connected to emotional memories from the time of the abuse. The survivor is reexperiencing the hopelessness he felt as a child. Differentiating between memories of old pain and what's actually happening in the present can sometimes lighten the survivor's despair.

The best antidote to hopelessness is the offer of hope. At his most low, the survivor needs to find something that inspires him, moves him, and renews his belief in life. Your faith in him can play a big part in keeping him going, but alone, it will not be enough. He needs to find a thread to keep him moving forward, even when he feels he's sinking.

Survivors need role models and examples that healing is possible. If he can identify with someone who's further along the road than he is, he'll be able to keep walking on that road.

If the survivor is sinking deeper and deeper into depression, make sure he's getting skilled support. Although it's natural to feel depressed when facing the enormity of healing, prolonged and deepening depression is a sign of serious distress. If you're feeling scared or are worried about the survivor's will to live, get professional help for *both of you*. And if the survivor is depressed to the point of being suicidal, turn to page 111.

How long does it take for a grown woman to progress from child to adult? Will she have to repeat her life year by year to make up for the dysfunction in her past? I get so frustrated by her. I don't know how to continue to be a spouse and a parent to her.

Survivors often need to go back and reexperience aspects of their childhood in the process of healing. Most survivors never had a chance to be children. Their sense of trust and innocence was destroyed by the abuse. They never had the freedom to explore the world as children. Many lived in families where they were forced to take on adult responsibilities at an early age. As a result, survivors grew up too fast, losing big chunks of experience and opportunities for learning along the way. Healing involves reclaiming those lost aspects of the self, picking up pieces that were left behind.

All of us can benefit from this kind of reintegration. We all have inner children; parts of ourselves that are silly or innocent or vulnerable; parts we may have split off to survive. Have you ever noticed yourself acting or sounding younger than usual? Looked in the mirror and seen an expression on your face you recognized from childhood? Felt like a ten-year-old when you played with your own children? These are traces of the inner child.

For some of us, the child within is readily accessible: we never lost touch with the younger parts of ourselves. For others, trauma, pain, and rigid conditioning forced the child underground: the inner child is split off and harder to reach. And in cases of extreme abuse, child parts sometimes split off entirely. This creative survival mechanism sometimes leads to the development of multiple personalities. (see page 136 for information on this unique coping strategy.)

Getting in touch with the inner child is an important part of the healing process for survivors. It's often the inner child who holds memories and feelings for the adult. Listening to the child often leads to the retrieval of memories—frequently painful or traumatic, sometimes pleasant. When the child's pain is recognized and released, the adult survivor is freed from using limiting survival strategies adopted in childhood. Getting in touch with the child can also help the survivor reclaim a sense of innocence and play.

On the outside, this reclaiming process can look pretty weird.

Survivors do a lot of regression—they begin feeling and acting like children, instead of like adults. For you, as a partner, this means that the grown-up you're used to relating to suddenly starts behaving and responding like a child. Sometimes the change is refreshing; your normally rigid partner is willing to laugh, play, and explore. If you're willing to jump right in there with your own childlike spirit, you can have a lot of fun. But other times, the changes can be extremely distressing. You want to be with a peer, and out of the blue you find yourself interacting with a frightened, withdrawn, or unmanageable child. What happened to the adult you were talking to five minutes ago?

The switch into a child state can be triggered by any number of things that remind the survivor of childhood—an angry tone of voice, the color of the shirt you're wearing, a body memory of abuse. The change often occurs when the survivor is scared, angry, upset, or sexually aroused. Switching can also be indicative of multiple personalities.

Watching a survivor in the middle of a regression looks like this: you're about to make love, are in the middle of an argument, or are getting ready to go out the door for work, and the survivor's face changes in front of your eyes. You suddenly find yourself looking at a seven-year-old or a toddler. The changes can be obvious or subtle. Simple, childlike language or shifts in body posture can be clues. If the survivor has regressed to babyhood, she may not be talking at all; she may be curled up sucking her thumb. At that moment, you are no longer interacting with an adult.

For the survivor, there's nothing inherently dangerous about regression. Feeling and acting like a child won't hurt the survivor (unless the child is feeling self-destructive and isn't being watched by a protective adult). In a safe environment, giving the child room to exist can be an informative, healing experience which can yield valuable information.

As a partner, though, you have different considerations. You thought the survivor was your peer and equal, and suddenly you have an extra child on your hands. You feel resentful, worried, and abandoned. This isn't what you signed up for. You don't know how to interact with her. You're scared and you feel alone.

There are two ways you can handle a regression: get in there and roll up your sleeves and go through it with her, or find a way for her to be safe (help her get grounded, enlist other support) and take care of yourself. You get to make the choice, and your answer may vary from day to day. Partners have different capacities and needs. It's important that you know yours. Ask yourself: "Am I willing to go through this regression with her? To help her through the memories that might emerge? Or do I need to go to work, make dinner, take care of myself?" "How scared am I?" "Is this something I can deal with right now?" It's essential that you know your limits. If you try to be there and you really don't want to, it will backfire on both of you. Set boundaries that reflect your real needs.

If you choose to be with the survivor while she's regressed, here are some guidelines: Talk to her just like you'd talk to a child of a comparable age. Reassure her that it's safe now to remember; that she'll be okay and that you'll stay with her. If she's having a flashback, listen and remember what she tells you. Ask her what she sees and feels. Ask her where she is, if someone else is with her. Sometimes she'll tell you what's going on; other times she won't want to. She may be experiencing feelings or body memories, with no words attached at all. At moments there's nothing you can do except be a witness to that kid: she's learning about her history, right there as she's cowering in the corner. Support her and love her, but give the child room to breathe. (See "Noah's Story" on page 258 for an example of a partner going through a flashback with a survivor.)

If you don't want to go through the survivor's regression with her, here are some things you can do to help her get grounded back into the present: Ask her to open her eyes, look at you, listen to the sound of your voice, walk around, describe what's in the room. Remind her where she is and who you are. Make her a cup of tea. Bring her a teddy bear and a blanket. Tuck her in. Read her a story. Rub her head. Call her therapist or someone from her support group so they can talk to her. (This can feel intrusive to the survivor if you haven't gotten permission to do so ahead of time.) Some therapists give clients a cassette tape in which they read a soothing story or lead the survivor in a relaxation exercise. Listening to it can help the survivor take care of herself. See if the survivor's therapist would be willing to make such a tape, if he or she hasn't already. Experiment. See what works best in bringing her back to the present. (What works well for one survivor can upset another.)

Fortunately, the process of reclaiming the inner child does not take as long as real growing up does. The survivor doesn't have to be four for a full year. Her puberty and adolescence won't span a decade. Things are integrated much faster than that. Initially, most survivors have little or no control over these changes in and out of the child state, but as time goes on, the survivor should be able to consciously bring herself in and out of the child state; to gain skills in taking care of the child herself. Eventually, the reparenting process should happen within the survivor: the adult part of her nurtures, protects, and takes care of the child.

Healing should involve an overall balance between regressive work and skill-building. It's just as important for the survivor to develop adult skills and abilities (building a support system, learning self-nurturing, developing communication skills) as it is for her to reclaim her inner child. A skilled counselor allows or encourages regression, but simultaneously teaches the survivor to reground in the present and come back to being an adult.

Remember that you're the survivor's partner, not her parent. Although there are ways you can support her or spend time with her when she's in her child-space, your role in life is not to be the primary caretaker of her inner children. There's only so much you can do. One partner explained her limits this way:

> Sometimes we take on too much, expect we should be able to do it all. I'm ambivalent myself. I want to be the "main" support, but I also want to have my own feelings of anger, frustration, and abandonment. It's been important for me to accept that her therapist is there for the constant, ongoing support. That frees me to be the partner, keeping myself and my needs in mind.

If the survivor is regressing a lot, help her find skilled people who can work with her and teach her skills in coming back on her own. Build a support team of people (friends, members of her support group, other survivors) who can stay with her when she's having trouble staying present as an adult.

Is my partner going to ALWAYS need me to go to the bathroom with her in the middle of the night?

No. Survivors needing this kind of extreme support are at a peak time of crisis. The survivor is reliving a time in her life when the nighttime was terrifying to her. Probably something happened to her in the middle of the night when she went to the bathroom as a child, and every time she goes to the bathroom she feels terrified that it will happen again. This may not be conscious, but it's why she can't let go of her partner's arm. When her partner goes with her, she feels safer, protected from her deepest fears. It's a lot like a child asking her mother to check the closet for the bogeyman. The survivor is reliving a particular developmental need, and like a child giving up a special blanky or a favorite stuffed bear, she will outgrow her need for this kind of security.

If the survivor needs this kind of support temporarily, and you can give it freely, that's great. If, on the other hand, you feel worn out and are tired of getting up every night, you can gradually wean her of her need for your physical presence. Maybe she could carry something with her, a safe object like a stuffed animal or a magic staff that she designs and creates herself. Designate a particular article of clothing, like your bathrobe or a big baggy shirt as a kind of armor that will protect her from bad things in the night. When she wears it, she's invincible. Install a series of nightlights or keep a light on in the hall. Be creative. Find something that works for her.

As she develops more of a sense of safety in herself, her ability to move around without fear will increase. In *The Courage to Heal Workbook* I taught survivors how to create a safe spot in their homes, a place untouched by threatening spirits and memories. This isn't possible for everyone to do initially, but gradually the survivor can learn to internalize a sense of safety. You can't be with her every minute of every day (nor would you want to) and she needs to learn to feel safe and protected on her own.

One of the best ways for survivors to gain a sense of safety is a self-defense class. (Call your local rape crisis center for classes that are sensitive to the needs of survivors.) Instruction in self-defense can decrease her fears and enable her to feel more confident taking care of herself.

Since he started getting memories, my lover has been unable to sleep at night. He's plagued by nightmares and wants me to hold him. I can't keep getting up with him every night. I'm exhausted.

Survivors have so many problems at night (insomnia, extreme insecurity, panic attacks) because so much sexual abuse takes place at night. Many survivors experience "night terrors": they can't sleep, wake up in the middle of the night sweating or screaming (sometimes at the very time they were raped or attacked), or need you to walk to the bathroom with them. When they do manage to sleep, they have nightmares full of violence and fragmented memories. Sleeplessness sometimes precedes a new memory or follows it. This can be very tough on you, but you need to understand that it is a natural outcome of having been sexually abused.

I encourage survivors to experiment with the ways they sleep—in a bed, in a reclining chair, in catnaps throughout the day, with a light on, with a hammer under their pillow, whatever helps them rest. Losing a few nights' sleep never killed anyone. Sometimes it's best not to fight it and to watch something boring on TV or to read a book (not about incest, mass murderers, or violence). You can also help the survivor check for some of the obvious reasons for insomnia—Did he read anything disturbing before bed? Did you two have a fight? Have trouble with sex before sleeping? Are you discussing sexual abuse right before his head hits the pillow? There can be physical reasons too—drinking caffeinated soft drinks or coffee, eating sugar or chocolate before bed. Sometimes exercise during the day can help tire the survivor's body so he can sleep better at night.

Sometimes a period of night terrors may just be a phase you have to live through. Like a child with nightmares or a child who gets up to go to the bathroom twice every night for a week after seeing a scary movie, you have to live with it and provide a sense of security and safety until the need for it diminishes. Here's one partner's creative solution:

I work at night. I come in when she's asleep. For years every time I came into the bedroom at night, she'd wake up with a scream. Not a pleasant welcome for me. I think that's fairly traumatic. We finally found one technique that helped. We had these Tibetan bowls. I'd ding them in the kitchen to let her know I was home.

If you can support the survivor by singing him a lullaby, bringing him a mug of warm milk, or by dinging Tibetan bowls, that's great. But if you can only get up with him twice a week, or on the weekends when you don't go to work, that's okay too. Sleep apart sometimes so you can get the rest you need. It's always best to give what you can give freely, without resentment and with love, than to overextend yourself and resent it later.

Of course, as a survivor, I prefer to have someone there for me if I can't sleep. If I wake up with a nightmare in the middle of the night, it helps tremendously for my partner to hear me out, reassure me, hold me, comfort me, and give me a reality check, but it's not absolutely essential. I've had nightmares and rotten nights' sleep when I've been alone, and I've gotten resourceful. I've taken to keeping a Walkman with fresh batteries and a relaxation tape next to the bed. I've gotten up and made myself a cup of chamomile tea. I've called a friend in another time zone (or one who's likely to be up for the same reasons). I prefer someone else to talk me down or out of it, but I have made it through some pretty hairy nights on my own. Survivors lived through the abuse. With creativity and support, they can live through some rough nights as well.

My lover repeatedly cuts himself until he draws blood. He's not actually trying to kill himself, but he keeps hurting himself, over and over. I'm completely freaked out by what he's doing. How can I stop him?

Many survivors consciously hurt themselves. Therapists call this self-mutilation. Survivors cut or burn themselves, punch their fists through glass, drive drunk and have car accidents, or otherwise put themselves in physical danger. Sometimes self-mutilation is done in secrecy and is kept hidden; other times the injuries are readily apparent. In all its forms, self-mutilation should be taken seriously. Don't try to deal with it alone.

Although it can be distressing to witness (and can be dangerous at times), self-injury is a survival skill. Sometimes it's a replication of the actual abuse. There's something about repeating an act of abuse, over and over, but this time controlling the injury and the pain themselves, that is oddly comforting to some survivors. They get to stop the pain whenever they want to. Their pain has an end and this time they're the one in control of it.

Other survivors were brainwashed and programmed to hurt or kill themselves. The abusers no longer have to injure the survivor; he's doing it to himself. He's playing out their programming and feels powerless to do otherwise. In order for him to stop, the self-destructive tapes have to be dismantled and replaced with life-affirming messages.

Other survivors injure themselves as a way of releasing some of the pain they feel on the inside. Their inner world is full of torment and unbearable suffering. It doesn't show on the outside. No one knows how bad they feel. Hurting themselves is a way of making the pain visible. Cutting becomes a cry for help. It speaks for the survivor: "Hey, I'm hurting in here. Won't you notice? Can't you do something to help me?"

Many survivors experience relief when they hurt themselves: it relieves some of the pressure. It's like letting some of the air out of a balloon that's so full it's about to burst. The physical pain hurts less than the emotional pain, and therefore it is a welcome distraction from the intense anguish the survivor feels on the inside.

Other survivors are so numb that they need the intense physical stimulation of self-mutilation to have any feelings at all. Making themselves bleed is life-affirming for them: it proves that they're human and alive.

Anger and self-hatred turned inward can also lead to self-mutilation. Cutting himself may be the only "safe" way the survivor knows to express his anger. Survivors also cut themselves when they feel scared or believe they "deserve to be punished": when they have sex, enjoy sex, talk about the abuse, have new memories, confront the perpetrator, or make some other breakthrough in their healing.

Self-mutilation can be an addictive habit that is hard to break. It is possible, however, to stop a pattern of self-abuse. The survivor has to want to stop, and will probably need professional help to do so.

The more a survivor gets in touch with his emotions and his anger, and learns to express them in other ways, the less compelled he'll be to cut or hurt himself. Emotional release work, getting feelings out through the body, are very effective antidotes to self-injury. So are writing, artwork, and other forms of creative expression. (One survivor began penning love notes to herself up and down her arm every time she had the urge to cut herself.)

Living with a survivor who hurts himself can be scary and confusing. Your response to what he's doing will fluctuate depending on the nature and severity of the injuries, but it's natural to feel frightened, powerless, and angry when faced with a survivor who intentionally injures himself. At times, you may question your commitment to the relationship. That's natural, too. Don't protect the survivor by keeping your feelings a secret. Tell him how you feel. Let him know how his actions are affecting you.

Self-mutilation is not usually life-threatening (the cuts are frequently superficial), but other times self-mutilation can cross the line into an attempt at suicide. (See page 111 for more on suicide.) If you're in an emergency situation and the survivor has hurt himself and needs to go to the hospital, call an ambulance or take him yourself. If the survivor comes to you and says, "I'm about to cut myself," ask for the weapon. Then call for help.

Get skilled help for the survivor so you can both feel safer. Then get help for yourself too. Don't isolate yourself or try to deal with this alone. Although you may feel ashamed or scared to talk about it, it's essential that you get support. (See page 162 for guidelines on choosing people to talk to.)

How can I deal with my fear of the survivor's suicidal tendencies?

Many survivors contemplate suicide. For some, the hopelessness and anguish involved in healing increase suicidal feelings which have always been there. Others feel suicidal for the first time as they confront the pain of the abuse. Still others have been programmed by their abusers to kill themselves at a particular point in time (if they disclose; when they reach a particular age). Survivors abused in satanic cults often become suicidal on trigger dates that correspond with specific cult rituals.

Suicidal feelings sometimes correspond to breakthroughs in a survivor's healing (confronting the offender, realizing she had an orgasm during the abuse, getting in touch with shame, dealing with new memories). Almost all survivors have moments when they'd rather be dead than face the abuse. Many contemplate suicide, but don't actually kill themselves. Tragically, others do, adding to the statistics of victims who don't make it.

Of course you want to do everything possible to prevent the survivor from committing suicide. One partner, who had skills in assessing suicide, described his experience:

> I had to do a suicide assessment with her. I asked, "Are you planning to hurt yourself? Do you feel like you could?" She admitted to me that she did. I asked, "Is there something available here that you could hurt yourself with?" She said she wanted to use razor blades on her wrists. I made her promise not to. I made her promise that if she felt suicidal again she would call me immediately. She promised. I felt lucky that I had the skills to evaluate the situation, but I was shocked and scared. I felt like I was losing a partner. There were a couple of months where I felt like I had lost her.

Since most of us aren't trained to deal with suicide, it's imperative that you seek help if the survivor starts talking about it. *Suicidal feelings and talk about suicide should be taken with complete seriousness. If the survivor is suicidal, don't try to deal with it alone. A suicidal survivor*

*needs resources beyond what you can offer. Get immediate professional atten-
tion and support for both of you.* If you don't already have a counselor,
call the operator or 911 and ask for the number of Suicide Prevention to help you locate resources in your area.

If the survivor has a therapist or support group, make sure the
counselor or support group members know that she's suicidal. Encourage the survivor to talk about her feelings to her therapist or
group, but if she isn't willing, talk to them anyway. This is one place
where it's okay to take the initiative without her permission. Her life
is at stake. You do whatever is necessary to keep her alive. That may
include hospitalization or other emergency measures.

Arrange a session for both of you with her therapist. Talk specifically about what each of you can do to prevent her suicide. See if
the survivor is willing to sign a no-suicide contract, in which she
agrees not to commit suicide until a certain designated time (until
she has contacted Suicide Prevention or her counselor, until her next
therapy appointment, until you come home from work and talk to
her). If it's possible, have her come up with the terms of the contract
herself. (*The Courage to Heal Workbook* has a sample no-suicide contract on page 70.)

When someone is going through the trauma of healing from
sexual abuse, it's natural to want to die. Her feelings are understandable, but her thinking is wrong: She believes her pain is so great that
only death can end it. That isn't true. If she survived the abuse, she
can survive the pain of healing, too.

Validate the survivor's feelings, but remind her of the difference
between feelings and actions. Tell her, "I know you're in terrible
pain right now, but it won't last forever. You feel like dying, but it's
important that you live. The abusers have taken enough victims already. Don't let them have you." With her therapist, help her come
up with a plan for dealing with panicky feelings. Together, assess
whether the survivor needs twenty-four-hour care.

As a partner, living with such a survivor is extremely frightening. It is terrifying to watch the person you love become increasingly
suicidal. You feel out of control (you are) and powerless to stop her
(ultimately, that's true too). Churning inside of you are tremendous
feelings of helplessness and rage. You probably feel an overwhelming fear of abandonment. Don't be afraid to let the survivor know
how you would feel if she killed herself. Tell her how scared and

upset you are. Tell her why you want her to live. Let her know how important she is to you. Your honest, human response may be a critical factor in her decision to live. And if you've reached your limit, and don't think you can take anymore, let the survivor know you won't be able to stay with her if she keeps suicide as an option.

It's imperative that you get your own support and help in coping with your feelings and in learning what you can and cannot do to help. Reach out. It's the most important thing you can do.

Ultimately, if someone is determined to commit suicide, no amount of support or intervention can stop her. If the survivor kills herself, it would be an immense tragedy and you would have to find a way to live with it. But it would not be your fault. You cannot control someone else's will to live or die.

MORE ABOUT
SEXUAL ABUSE

"When you get involved with someone at the beginning of dealing with incest, you just don't know what the hell you're getting into. Everyone is different. No one's going to heal in exactly the same way. I could tell you, 'This is what happened to me and my partner,' but you might experience something very different."

"I was panicked when she first started getting memories. Then it calmed down to scared."

"I've actually had the thought, 'Jesus Christ, if every memory you've had has really happened to you, I'm amazed you survived and are still alive.' "

Why did it take twenty years for my lover's memories of child physical and sexual abuse to surface?

One of the most powerful and effective ways children survive abuse is to block it out, to push the awareness of the experience away. Children actually forget the abuse happened; they store it away in a part of themselves that isn't available to their conscious minds. This isn't universally true; many children never forget what happened to them. But many survivors grow to adulthood with no memory of the abuse. They live with the effects of the abuse, but have no idea why they're scared of being touched, cut off from their feelings, or fearful of the people they love. Then ten or twenty years later, these repressed childhood memories surface, often creating havoc in their lives (and yours).

It may be difficult for you to accept the idea that memories can suddenly surface "out of thin air," but the process of recovering traumatic memories years after the original trauma is a well-documented psychological phenomenon. No one knows exactly why one person never forgets, one waits five years to remember, and a third remembers after twenty-five.

For some survivors, having distance from the abuse (and the abuser) and a feeling of safety are prerequisites to remembering. Others remember when their lives are in crisis and coming undone. One man said, "It was like a closet that was full to bursting. The door just couldn't hold anymore."

Memories can be triggered by a number of factors: a TV show, an article in the newspaper, a movie like *The Color Purple* or *Nuts,* news of a child abused down the street, a friend's story. A simple sensory trigger, such as the sound of a dog barking (if a dog was barking at the time of the abuse), smelling bourbon on someone's breath, or being awakened in the middle of the night, can send a survivor into a nightmare state—and bring back memories of early abuse.

The death of the abuser or another significant family member can be a trigger, too. The survivor is no longer at risk; the abuser can no longer hurt him. He remembers after his mother dies because the disclosure can no longer hurt her. Any major loss or transition can bring up feelings of earlier losses—the loss of innocence, the loss of trust, the loss of self in childhood.

HOW MEMORIES SURFACE

Memories are stored in the body, and physical touch can bring them to the surface. You touch the survivor in a particular way and he goes numb, disappears, or thinks you're his brother on top of him in the narrow bed he slept in as a child. Survivors remember during massages, bodywork (therapies that integrate touch and movement), physical exercise, or in the course of other body changes, like losing or gaining a lot of weight. (For more on flashbacks, see page 187.)

The feeling of having his body compromised, in pain, and out of control while undergoing medical testing, surgery, or anesthesia, can bring back similar feelings of childhood. So can visits to the dentist: for survivors who were orally raped, going to the dentist can be a terrible trauma. Visits to the gynecologist or proctologist can also evoke painful memories.

Parenting is evocative of our own childhood; when we have children, we recall more from our own growing up years. Many men, in particular, seek out therapy when they're about to become fathers; they're afraid of the myth that sexually abused boys inevitably grow up to be child molesters (this is *not* true). For a woman, being pregnant can be a trigger: her body is changing and the changes are out of her control, an experience that echoes back to abuse. Survivors remember abuse when their child reaches the age they were when they were first abused, reaches the age of the original offender, or is also abused. A daughter turns four and her mother starts having flashbacks. A man abused as a boy by his fourteen-year-old cousin starts to have memories when his son reaches puberty. Or he remembers so he can come forward and protect a child in the next generation who is at risk from the same abuser.

When survivors break an addiction to alcohol, cigarettes, drugs, sex, or eating, they often come face to face with memories during early sobriety. If they're victimized as adults—raped, robbed, battered, or fired from a job—earlier times they felt powerless can come to the surface.

Aging can be another trigger. We're all aging, but there are certain times when aging means a loss of power and status. Dealing with the associated feelings—loss of control, self-esteem, and dignity —can resonate deeply with childhood abuse.

There is no right way or time for a survivor to remember. Memories can't be forced, and when they surface—whether it's after five, ten, or thirty years—that's the right time to deal with them.

As a partner, you'll probably have times you wish the memories would go back where they came from (and often, the survivor would agree with you), but I believe it's worthwhile to know our history. I hated remembering the abuse, I hated the way it turned my world upside down, but I liked the fact that my crazy experience of life suddenly made sense.

It's likely that you will go through times when you struggle to accept and believe the survivor's memories. Do what you can to learn about the process of remembering so you can gradually come to believe and support him. Survivors have been denied and discredited most of their lives; if you want to be supportive, you'll need to find a way to work through your own denial and disbelief.

Do the memories have to be fully remembered in order for the survivor to heal?

No. It's possible to heal from the effects of the abuse without remembering the details of what happened. Some survivors gain complete recall of the abuse; others never get more than a funny feeling in the pit of their stomachs. The crucial thing is for the survivor to put together whatever clues she has so she can accept the fact that the abuse took place. These clues can include bits of family history, memory gaps, things that trigger her in the present, effects of abuse that show up in her life, reactions to other survivors' stories, as well as bits of visual, auditory, olfactory, or body memory. For each survivor, the pieces of the puzzle will be different.

Survivors who have a lot of visual memory (pictures of the actual abuse) often feel inundated and overwhelmed by the images. Those who don't have pictures wish they did; they minimize or negate the clues they do have because they are not visual. We've all been conditioned in a visual culture; we believe picture memory is the only kind that really counts. It isn't.

The important thing is for survivors to eventually reach a point where they can say, "Yes, it happened. The effects are imprinted in my life. I'm going to accept the fact that I was abused and make a commitment to heal, even if I never remember the specifics." Memory is not a prerequisite to healing. Willingness, determination, and courage are.

As a partner, it can be harder to believe the abuse if there isn't proof in the form of clear memories. We've all watched "Perry Mason" and "Columbo": we know the kind of evidence you need to accuse someone of a crime. You're hesitant to accuse your father-in-law of something that happened twenty years ago because the survivor had a sketchy dream or a panic attack. Yet that's all you have to go on. Unfortunately, child sexual abuse (especially when it happened twenty years ago) doesn't usually leave much in the way of concrete evidence.

It's natural to have doubts; but ultimately, if you want to be her intimate supporter, you need to find a way to believe the abuse happened, even if the survivor never recovers another memory. The survivor is full of her own doubts; she doesn't need yours to deal with, too.

If you're struggling with the issue of insufficient proof, stop waiting for that one, conclusive memory. Look instead to the circumstantial evidence: the effects of abuse (outlined on page 17); the similarity between your struggles and the ones you're reading about in this book. Reread the section on "Denial" (page 51). Read through the partners' stories (page 243). Their words and struggles may give you the validation you need.

Why do abusers get away with it?

Abusers get away with it because of the massive denial of sexual abuse in our culture. Until recently (and still in some quarters), sexual abuse has been seen as something extremely rare or basically benign. The sexual abuse and even torture of children is regularly rationalized, justified, and excused.

Although our society has begun to say no to physical and sexual abuse, that "no" is relatively recent.[1] In many states, the legal penalty for sexual abuse is nothing more than a slap on the wrist. Child abusers often plea bargain and receive suspended sentences or probation. Many are not even forced into treatment. The punishment for raping children does not fit the crime.

Prosecuting child sex abuse cases is difficult, and in many ways, is becoming more difficult. There is a backlash in the court system, an outright battle about how child sex abuse cases should be tried.[2] The testimony of children is still being discredited in many states, and the court process itself continues to add to the trauma experienced by many young victims. Children are being encouraged to tell, to talk about the abuse, but when they do, the social service and judicial systems that intervene are often woefully inadequate, and sometimes harmful.

Why do abusers get away with it? Because abusers are respected members of the community; because they're breadwinners and their families rely on them; because they're mothers and "mothers don't hurt their own children"; because "a man's home is his castle"; because no one wanted to see it: the neighbor turned away, the family friend didn't want trouble, the teacher worried about her job, the pediatrician covered it up, the neighbor wanted to keep the peace, the minister told them to pray, the social worker was overloaded, and the grocery store owner didn't know what to do.

---

[1] For more on the history of child sexual abuse see *The Best Kept Secret* by Florence Rush, *Father-Daughter Incest* by Judith Herman, the introduction to *I Never Told Anyone* by Ellen Bass, and *The Conspiracy of Silence* by Sandra Butler.

[2] For more on the current legal battles over child sex abuse, read *The Battle and the Backlash* by David Hechler. *On Trial* by Billie Wright Dziech, *Home Front* by Louise Armstrong, and *By Silence Betrayed* by John Crewsdon. See the bibliography for details.

WHY DO ABUSERS GET AWAY WITH IT?

Why do abusers get away with it? Because "it's not nice to talk about such things," because "children exaggerate," "she must have asked for it," "little girls are seductive," "it doesn't happen to boys," and "it only happens in those other kinds of homes." That's why.

When you think about the impact of sexual abuse, about the lost potential, the terrible grief, the price we pay as individuals and as a society, it is really unthinkable that we allow abuse to continue. Yet we do. For the status quo to change (a new generation of victims every ten years), we need to do more than just treat the survivors who've already been abused (although of course that's essential). We need to take direct action in changing our basic institutions and attitudes. If we don't, the question "why do they get away with it?" will be asked by our grandchildren and great-grandchildren as they wonder why it happened to them, too.

I do not understand how someone can physically or sexually abuse another human being, especially another family member. I just don't get it.

I don't either. It's one of the most agonizing questions I live with. Accepting the reality of abuse has made me question all the assumptions I've had about what makes us human. Anne Frank, when facing the Nazis, wrote in her journal that "People are basically good at heart." Doing this work has made me wonder.

Why do some people use their pain as a motivation to create beauty while others callously destroy human life? Why does one survivor commit suicide when another makes it out of that same hellhole alive? Why does one survivor face the abuse and another continue to deny it? How can a father rape his own daughter? A mother torture her own son? Or as one partner simply said, "How could anyone do something so evil?"

Intellectually, I could sit here and lay out the standard answers about why these things happen. I could talk about the things that enabled the child to survive: the grandmother who loved the child, the spiritual connection the child made when she sang in the church choir. I could write about the father's unresolved pain and trauma, and speculate about whether he felt pain when he went to his daughter's bed. I could tell you that abusers abuse because they were abused as children, but that wouldn't explain why so many survivors of torture, unbelievably horrible torture, never abuse anyone, and in fact go on to become protectors of children. I could talk about the political and moral climate of our culture, a culture in which child sexual abuse thrives. I could talk about the history of child sexual abuse and document the institutionalized abuse of children.[1] But none of these things for me explains the simple human act: how does a father rape his daughter at night and get up able to face himself in the morning?

For me, every question raises another, more impenetrable ques-

---

[1] Read *The Best Kept Secret* by Florence Rush, *The Conspiracy of Silence* by Sandra Butler. *Father-Daughter Incest* by Judith Herman, and the introduction to *I Never Told Anyone* by Ellen Bass for a historical and political perspective on child sexual abuse. See the bibliography for details.

tion: Why? Why do we live in a world where this is happening? Why don't we respect and protect our children? Why have so many people I love been sexually abused? These are questions you will face in a thousand ways.

Being intimately involved with a survivor will make you ask questions that challenge your deepest beliefs and values. No one can hand you a list of right answers. You will have to wrestle with these questions in your own heart and mind until you find a truth you can live with.

My partner despairs that he'll never get over the abuse because he can't imagine forgiving his mother for what she did to him. He feels stuck and I feel stuck with him. What can he do?

Forgiveness, although frequently recommended by well-meaning (and not so well-meaning) people, is not a necessary stage of the healing process. Although some survivors naturally reach a place of forgiveness after moving through the other stages of healing, *it is not necessary to forgive the abuser in order to heal.* Forgiveness is a personal choice and a personal experience, but it's not the end of the healing process or the ultimate goal of healing.

The important thing is for the survivor to come to a place of resolution in his relationship with the abuser. Resolution may include setting clear limits and boundaries, suing the abuser in court, cutting ties with the abuser, or even coming to a place of reconciliation. But it does not necessarily include forgiveness.

People often say to me, "But if you don't forgive, you're destined to walk around bitter and angry for the rest of your life." I don't believe that. It hasn't been my personal experience. I haven't forgiven my grandfather for sexually abusing me, and I don't feel embittered. I hate what he did to me. I wish he hadn't done it. But I don't walk around seething all the time. He's dead now, and in my mind, he seems very distant and far away. I've moved on with my life and my healing. I rarely think about him anymore.

One of the things survivors hear most frequently (again, often from well-meaning supporters) is that they should forgive because the abuser was abused as a child.[1] That argument doesn't hold water with me, either. As one survivor put it:

> I'm sick of hearing that crap about abusers being abused.
> I was abused and I haven't turned around and done it to
> someone else. Having it done to you is no excuse.

Even when abusers deny the abuse or don't acknowledge that it was wrong, survivors are still expected to forgive. As one survivor put it so well:

---

[1] See *Banished Knowledge* by Alice Miller for an analysis of this phenomenon.

Why should I forgive someone who's never acknowledged he hurt me and never said he's sorry? Until he takes responsibility for his actions, I can't even begin to think about forgiveness.

Many survivors struggle particularly hard with the pressure to forgive because of their religious beliefs. Christian beliefs (and many New Age spiritual beliefs as well) stress forgiveness as a virtue. If you or the survivor are struggling with the belief that forgiveness is a prerequisite to healing, there's been some excellent writing coming out of the Christian community which clarifies and sheds new light on the interplay between sexual abuse and forgiveness. I recommend these books highly for anyone having trouble reconciling their sense of outrage with their belief system.[2]

The clearest, most heartfelt response to the forgiveness question came in a letter Ellen Bass and I received in response to *The Courage to Heal*. Its author captures the essence of the forgiveness debate better than anyone else I've heard. Pay particular attention to the way she signs her letter. Ask yourself if she sounds like a bitter person:

Dear Ellen and Laura,

I had been standing in the bookstore for an hour facing the shelves of self-help books that had so many titles even my trifocals couldn't sort out the plethora of advice available. I was still raw from last month's graduation from the treatment center. My medallion with the Serenity Prayer on it was still warm from the energy infused by my peers in Therapy Group as they passed it around while they said goodbye to me.

I needed help but couldn't locate the books my counselor recommended and was about to give up on them, when my husband pointed out *The Courage to Heal* and I added that to the

---

[2] Malcolm Burson et al., *Discerning the Call to Social Ministry: An Alban Institute Case Study in Congregational Outreach*. New York, 1990. You can order copies by sending $10.95 to The Alban Institute, 4125 Nebraska Ave. NW, Washington, DC, 20016. Also read *Sexual Violence: The Unmentionable Sin* by Marie Fortune, and *Slayer of the Soul: Child Sexual Abuse and the Catholic Church* by Stephen Rossetti. Both are listed in the bibliography.

stack of books I had chosen with titles that so seductively offered to make me whole.

That was the best thing I've done in years! Both of you and your "courageous women" have been right here with me ever since. I love you all for setting me free from a bondage that had held me for nearly half a century . . . I DON'T HAVE TO FORGIVE MY FATHER! My counselors agreed that I had intellectually forgiven him but they wanted me to sound out good things about him and dredge up any times when I had had love for him, but try as I would, I wasn't comfortable with that approach. It didn't feel right for me—mainly because I have maintained for two generations that incest is *unforgivable*.

When I agreed to enter treatment for my alcoholism, I didn't know you couldn't select just alcohol-related problems to deal with. I didn't realize the alcohol issues would trigger an overwhelming number of traumas to be exposed for my consideration! Now I realize the incest issue is looming larger for me than the one of alcohol addiction. My new vulnerability makes me shiver and want to curl up and protect myself, but my reborn anger and resentment overrides that and fuels my need to rethink my life and move on.

I thank you for my new freedom. I can heal now . . . I *am* healing already. You would faint and fall in if you could see this overweight, 58 yr. old granny leaping and shouting to the skies, "WhaaHOO! I don't have to forgive the old fucker after all!"

And then she signs her letter: "Yours in the newness of life."

I'm not antifeminist, but I'm getting tired of all this feminist talk. Why the increase?

Feminism, at its core, is a movement which has identified the oppression of women and helped women reclaim their power. Feminism directly challenges the institutions which have kept women "in their place," and has consistently fought for women's equality and right to determine their own lives. The struggle to stop violence against women has been led by feminists, who are responsible for bringing issues like rape, pornography, sexual abuse, battery, and child abuse into public awareness. Survivors would still be suffering in silence, with no resources or information to help them, if it were not for the feminist movement. Everyone concerned with the welfare of survivors owes a huge debt to the feminist movement. None of us would be "healing" or "reclaiming our lives" today if it weren't for the groundbreaking efforts of feminists.

As the survivor gets in touch with her pain, and realizes that millions of others have been hurt as well, it's natural for her to get angry. The best thing she can do with that anger is focus it and direct it back out into the world that hurt her. She may be realizing that the problem of violence against women and children is not an individual sorrow; it is systemic: our culture allows it to continue. Until the systems we live by—judicial, legislative, familial, educational—are overhauled, women and children will continue to be abused. When a survivor realizes the extent of abuse in our culture, and starts to look at its implications (a huge portion of the population trained to be passive victims), it's natural to become politicized.

I strongly encourage survivors, both male and female, to take a political stance against abuse. I hope you will do so, too. It's the only way we're going to stop abuse.

As a male partner of a female survivor, however, it can be disconcerting for your partner to start talking about the evils of men. One partner explained:

> She's become much more aware of the portrayal of violence toward women in the media. She's very angry about men and women in the world and their roles in the world, and men's responsibility for violence, pestilence, and war.

Men don't sit very well with her. She thinks of them as the reason for most of the ills in the world. And I tend to fall into that category of being a man.

You may also be feeling personally threatened by the fact that the survivor is asserting her independence, getting angry, and standing up for herself. Although you may not be used to this, it's an essential part of her healing. She's getting in touch with her own sense of power. Instead of feeling threatened, see if you can find ways to support her. Ask yourself, "Have I had more of the power and control in this relationship?" "Have I benefited from being involved with someone who doesn't stand up to me?" "What would it feel like to give up some of my power?" "Am I willing to?" "Why or why not?"

Many men feel relieved to give up the deeply ingrained sexual roles they've been taught to play. Not all men want to be dominant and in control.[1] As the balance of power shifts in your relationship, you'll be free to explore other aspects of yourself that have been buried underneath your role as "the competent, in-control, rational man." You may also feel deeply relieved that there's something you can do to make up for the violence and abuse other men have inflicted. To a caring, sensitive man, it is painful to witness the damage that's been caused by other men. Many male partners in workshops have said they feel deeply ashamed of their maleness. "When I realized the things men did to children," one partner said, "I didn't want to be a man anymore."

With the encouragement of the other men in the group, this man joined a men's antiviolence group that did education and consciousness-raising work. He ran a series of workshops for young men on college campuses to help eliminate date rape. He joined the survivor in her desire to fight back, and in the process became the kind of man he could be proud of. Through his actions, he became a feminist.

The goal of this work is to stop abuse, not just to put a band-aid on individual hurts. When you love someone whose healing is lead-

---

[1] For some literature on the emerging "men's movement," see "About Men" in the bibliography.

ing her to challenge abuse in the world, you either support her in that effort or you stand in the way. If you really want to support the survivor's healing, join her in fighting back.

How should I handle the comment "You're just like all the other men"?

The answer to this question depends on the kind of man you are. Unfortunately, when women make sweeping generalizations about how men are, some men do fit into the stereotype—domineering, controlling, oppressive, and violent. As one male partner explained, it's part of the culture:

> Why are men violent? My lover and I went to see the movie *Born on the Fourth of July*. That's why men become abusers. Men are born to go to war and kill. But men are not born killers. They don't come out of their momma's womb ready to rape and kill. It's not like that. It's programming like everything else. Sometimes I have to remind myself of that.

When someone has been consistently hurt by one gender, it's easy to assume that all members of that gender share the same characteristics. (Women receive this kind of blanket judgment, too.) It's a form of self-protection, a way of never being vulnerable to the same level of hurt again. Like any other bias, it has its roots in a painful process of childhood conditioning.

When the survivor tells you, "You're just like all the other men," look first to see if there's any truth in what she's saying. (For more on how to do this, see page 95.) If you still feel unjustly accused or unfairly lumped in with a kind of man or a type of behavior that you don't identify with, point out the ways you're different from the men who have abused her. Tell her it hurts you to be lumped in with a type of man you've worked hard not to be. Let her know you don't like those kinds of men either.

If the survivor doesn't like or trust men, and you're a man, you might also want to ask yourself why you're in a relationship with someone who dislikes men. It may be that you're harboring some internalized self-hatred of your own. This may be a time when you want to do some positive affirming of your maleness. (See "About Men" in the bibliography for some resource ideas.)

When a survivor has been hurt over and over by men, it's natural for her to come to the conclusion that men are hurtful and dangerous. If you don't fit her stereotype of a violent or domineering man, you may be the first man she's ever met who isn't that way. Time and exposure to a different kind of man will gradually break through her assumption that all men are the same. Through her relationship with you, she will have a chance to learn through first-hand experience that individual men are different and can be trusted. That's a powerful gift you can offer.

What are the results of cult abuse? Will my lover ever find his soul again?

Cult abuse has far-reaching effects on its victims.[1] In addition to the problems most survivors of sexual abuse and incest already experience, cult abuse survivors also have to deal with the results of brainwashing, severe intimidation, extreme humiliation, sensory deprivation, starvation, forced drug experiences, extreme torture, and the trauma of witnessing or being forced to participate in ritual murders or abuse of animals or other children. They are told their participation in these crimes is voluntary; that they are evil and have no recourse but to join the cult. Many child-victims are born and raised by parents who are already in the cult; they are systematically indoctrinated into cult membership from the time they are babies.

Cult survivors often blot out the experience by escaping into alcohol, drugs, and dissociation. Many cope with the severity of the trauma by developing multiple personalities (see page 136).

Victims who escape the cult (many do not) are often given posthypnotic suggestions which tell them to commit suicide, "go crazy," or return to the cult, rather than talk about their experiences. When cult survivors succeed in breaking the grip of mind control and disclose the abuse, they are rarely believed because of the extreme nature of these crimes. No one wants to believe that children are forced to kill babies, that adults bury children in coffins and tell them Satan is coming for them.[2] Many therapists, law enforcement personnel, judges, and lawyers prefer to believe that cult abuse survivors are suffering from hallucinations; that their memories are merely fantasies. This makes disclosure even more traumatic.

Because of the injunctions against telling and the effects of mind control, cult experiences are often the last to surface in a remembering process. Many cult survivors remember incidents of incest or child sexual abuse first, but are left with the sense that their memo-

---

[1] Thanks to Susan Schrader and Paul Kimmell for their excellent training on cult survivors at the Male Survivor Conference in Tuscon, Arizona in the fall of 1990. Their clarity and expertise helped me shape this essay.
[2] Satanic cults, in which members worship Satan, are only one of the types of cults that torture and abuse children. There are other cults, who commit similar crimes, whose practices are not connected to satanism.

ries don't sufficiently explain their feelings. They continue to be plagued by dreams of ritual violence. For many, this leads to memories of cult abuse.[3]

Many adult cult survivors continue suffering from the effects of mind control. They identify with the cult and see themselves as evil or bad. The core feeling is that there is no escape; that members of the cult are watching their every thought and move. For survivors to make progress in healing, these bonds of mind control must be broken.

Healing from the effects of satanic cult abuse is similar to healing for any survivor. There are some crucial differences, however. Sometimes the survivor will already have done a lot of work on incest or other sexual abuse before the cult memories surface. Because of the intensity of cult memories, the survivor may go right back to the crisis stage of healing.[4] The level of terror cult survivors experience is usually greater than that of other sexual abuse survivors. Because of the cult's programming, cult survivors often struggle with stronger and more long-lasting self-destructive impulses than other survivors. Due to early indoctrination into satanism and other belief systems, spiritual concerns frequently play a crucial role in healing. And in cases of intergenerational cult abuse, continued interactions with the family or the cult are dangerous for the survivor and should be avoided.

It can also be harder for a cult survivor to believe that the abuse happened because of its extreme nature. Since believing the abuse happened is crucial to moving through the rest of the stages of the healing process, progress may be slowed. It may also be harder for you as the partner to believe the survivor's memories. Cult experiences are horrifying and can seem unbelievable.

The first time I heard about cult abuse, I got sick and threw up

---

[3] Upon learning about cult abuse, many survivors think about the level of pain they're experiencing and wonder if they, too, were abused in a cult. On reading about cults, you may wonder the same thing yourself. New memories do sometimes reveal cult involvement. But more often, additional memories have to do with another perpetrator or a yet unrevealed incident of abuse, not abuse in a cult. Not everyone who wonders if they were abused in a cult was.

[4] Just because your partner is dealing with cult abuse doesn't necessarily mean he or she won't be able to function (although sometimes, it will). Many cult survivors have developed coping skills which enable them to function in their daily lives even though they are dealing with extreme trauma. (See "Virginia's Story" on page 293.)

for three days. My body felt polluted; I couldn't get the pictures out of my mind and body. I didn't want to believe the things I had heard; I was sorry I had asked. But after three days of trying to push the images away, I realized that if I wanted to support survivors, I had to get past my own shock, horror, and denial and come to terms with the fact that these things can, and do, happen. I need a lot of support to do that, and you will too.

Not all partners have to struggle to believe the cult abuse occurred. Noah had a different experience:

> I didn't have any trouble believing the cult stuff. At that point, after all we'd gone through with the sexual abuse, I would have believed anything. It was kind of like climbing a ladder. I didn't know much about violence. I didn't grow up in a violent family. But then I met my partner and she said she was beaten all the time, so I started to get used to that idea. Fathers and mothers beat their children, hit them, throw them across the room. She was raped. That was another level. Then we found out she'd been sexually abused as a child, as an infant. It was not hard for me to believe it at that point. I'd been around a lot more survivors. I'd heard a lot about sexual abuse and I'd seen how common it was. Then we found out about the ritual abuse. We went to a workshop for ritual survivors. It was just another step up the ladder.

If you are a partner of someone abused in a cult, you are facing an extensive healing process. Supporting a cult survivor will be a trial of your love and perseverance, although it is possible to vary your level of involvement depending on your own needs. (See "Noah's Story" on page 258 and "Virginia's Story" on page 293 for two very different examples of partners' involvement.) There may be times you wonder if you're up to the task; times you consider leaving the relationship. It's understandable that you would have those feelings. If you're feeling overwhelmed and uncertain about your ability to stay in the relationship, see page 87.

There is still a lot of disbelief among professionals about cult abuse, but training is now available in many parts of the country. More and more therapists are learning how to work with the special needs of cult survivors. Resources continue to grow. Cult survivors themselves are organizing, putting out newsletters, sponsoring educational forums, retreats, and resources for each other. (See the "Ritual Abuse" section of the bibliography for a list of books and organizations.) It's essential that practical and emotional support for partners be developed, too.

What are multiple personalities?

When children go through extreme childhood trauma (cult abuse, sadistic torture, witnessing a killing, severe sexual abuse), they sometimes develop multiple personalities.[1] When a child can't endure the pain he's experiencing and can't physically get away, he forms a new personality to contain the pain and survive the experience. This splitting-off process can happen once or many times. As a creative way of coping and surviving extreme abuse, the capacity to create new personalities is a formidable testimony to the resourcefulness of the human mind and spirit.

The development of new personalities (sometimes called "alters") is a form of dissociation. Dissociation means splitting off from yourself; it's something all of us do sometimes. Have you ever driven down the highway and suddenly reached your exit without being aware of how you got there? Asked your "conscience" or your "inner wisdom" what to do? Been in touch with your inner child? Heard the critical voice of a parent who wasn't really there? These are common forms of dissociation.

Dissociation exists on a continuum. At one end of the continuum is full awareness. As you move along the continuum, you have dulling or tuning out; then repression, the choice to put a painful experience aside. Next comes dissociation, a physiological response to sensory overload: the body's automatic response to stimulation it can't absorb or assimilate. Abused children (and people in wars or car accidents) often describe seeing their experiences from a distance: "I felt like I was up on the ceiling." "It was like I was standing far away, off in the paddy, watching myself shoot the gun." This is dissociation. As you move further along the continuum, dissociation becomes more severe. At the far end, distinct personalities split off to hold and contain the trauma. It is this more dramatic end of the spectrum that has been popularized in movies and books such as *Sybil, The Three Faces of Eve,* and *When Rabbit Howls.* Most survivors with multiple personalities have much less drama in their lives.

---

[1] Conversations with Ellen Bass, Robin Moulds, and Jim Struve were integral to the development of this essay. So was Susan Schrader and Paul Kimmell's excellent training on cult survivors at the Male Survivor Conference in Tucson, Arizona in the fall of 1990. Thank you all.

Most survivors talk to their inner children or inner parts; that doesn't necessarily mean they have multiple personalities. To be diagnosed with multiple personalities, survivors have to be further along the continuum, where the internal boundaries between different parts are less permeable.

Survivors with multiple personalities are often high functioners with many talents. Each personality holds a part of the self, a certain set of memories, a piece of the survivor's history. Different alters can have different skills and abilities: one might be an accomplished painter; another might be good at math. One personality might be suicidal or violent; another angry; another seductive and sexual. One might have asthma; another might not. Alters can be women or men, children or adults, and can have different sexual orientations.

For survivors with multiple personalities to heal, each alter has to go through a healing process. By learning to communicate with each other, alters begin to share the information and experiences they carry for the survivor. Each part has its place in the system: even alters that are self-destructive or violent serve a function. Each personality has played a role in protecting the survivor; everyone takes part in healing, too.

When you first learn that a survivor has multiple personalities, it's easy to feel frightened and overwhelmed. You may panic and want to run away. Allow yourself to have those feelings. But take some time to learn about what (and who) you're dealing with.[2] A diagnosis of multiple personalities doesn't mean the survivor is going to radically change; it just means there's a name for what you've already been experiencing. If things seem chaotic now, they won't necessarily stay that way. Over time, the survivor will learn to have more control over the switching process.

For some partners, finding out a survivor has multiple personalities is actually a relief: your relationship has been full of crazy surprises and you've had the funny feeling that you were interacting with more than one person. Now you have an explanation.[3]

---

[2] *United We Stand: A Book for People with Multiple Personalities* by Eliana Gil can give you an excellent place to start. See "Multiple Personalities" in the bibliography for this and other resources.

[3] Not all partners have this sense of recognition. See "Virginia's Story" on page 293 for a different point of view.

MULTIPLE PERSONALITIES

Although you aren't the survivor's therapist, you will probably have a chance to get to know some of his alters (if you don't know them already). The key to interacting with different personalities is to be with whoever is in front of you. Relate to them as people. Treat them the way you would anyone else—with respect, consideration, and interest. Learning about the survivor's other personalities can be clarifying, scary, exciting, sad, and even fun at times. You may get children you didn't know you had; lovers you weren't aware of.

Unfortunately, there's been a lot of hysteria in the media about multiple personalities recently. It's being treated like the exotic disease-of-the-week on TV and in the popular press. It's easy to be scared by what you read or to be misinformed by sensationalized reporting. This is one reason you need competent, professional help.

If you're with a survivor who has multiple personalities, you're with someone who's suffered very severe abuse. As a result, the healing process is going to take many years. Expect that you and the survivor will need long-term professional help, both individually and together. This is not something you should try to deal with alone.

The diagnosis of multiple personalities is still controversial; lots of mental health professionals don't believe the phenomenon exists. In many communities, there are minimal or inadequate resources; it may be hard for you to find a therapist with the skills and training to help. Be an advocate in getting the survivor the services he or she needs. Keep looking and fighting for the quality of help the survivor deserves. Urge your local mental health center to get training on multiple personalities so they can provide skilled, professional services. Fight your insurance company if you have to.

People with multiple personalities have also begun to organize their own grass-roots networks, support groups, and resources. Through one of these organizations, it may be possible to get referrals or to connect with other partners in your situation. (See the Resource section for more.)

My wife was sexually abused by her therapist. She blames herself and says she should have stopped it. She's been really depressed since it happened, but won't go to anyone else for counseling. I'm furious. She went for help and this guy screwed her over. He doesn't even acknowledge he did anything wrong. I want to stop him. Is there any legal recourse we can take?

Sexual abuse by therapists is a serious and unacceptable form of exploitation that is just beginning to be addressed. There have been books written,[1] laws passed, conferences held, and guidelines established by many of the professional associations that oversee counselors. These changes are a huge step in the right direction, but many survivors have already been, and still are being, sexually exploited and abused by therapists.

Because of the power imbalance inherent in the therapeutic relationship, it is critical that therapists, bodyworkers, religious counselors, doctors, and others working in a healing capacity do not have intimate or sexual relationships with their clients, patients, parishioners, or congregants. This is a boundary that should be respected with anyone who comes for help, but it is even more important for survivors. For a counselor to participate in an intimate or sexual relationship with a client who has been sexually abused is to directly duplicate the dynamics of the abuse—someone with more power manipulating the vulnerability of a survivor to fulfill his or her own needs.[2]

For many survivors, the relationship they establish with a counselor is the first caring nonsexual relationship they've ever had. It's essential that it stay that way. Even if the survivor is sexually attracted to the counselor or falls in love with the counselor, it is the counselor's job to maintain professional boundaries.

Survivors who have been sexually abused by a counselor often feel ashamed and responsible. If they were attracted to the counselor or liked the special attention they got, they view the abuse as an

---

[1] See "Abuse by Helping Professionals" in the bibliography.
[2] Not all abuse by therapists is sexual; there are also breaches of confidentiality and emotional boundaries.

"affair," and mistakenly believe it was their fault. Because they trusted and depended on the counselor, it is hard for them to name the experience as abuse or to hold the counselor responsible. This mirrors their response to the original abuse.

Once the survivor identifies the experience as abuse, she now has two sets of problems to resolve: the original abuse which has not been dealt with and the new layer of abuse by the therapist. Most survivors who've been abused by a therapist are reluctant to trust a therapist again, so many are stuck trying to deal with the double victimization without adequate support and advocacy.

As the partner of someone abused by a counselor, you may find yourself feeling jealous and angry, wondering if the survivor had a part in creating the sexual relationship with her therapist. You, too, may be inclined to view the whole thing as an affair in which you were betrayed. Remind yourself that the relationship between therapist and client is not an equal one. The survivor's job was to be vulnerable; to trust her therapist. The therapist manipulated that trust for his or her own selfish needs (and probably took money for it, besides!). That's hardly a reciprocal affair. *When sex happens between a therapist and a client, the fault and the responsibility always lie with the therapist.*

You may also respond to the news that the survivor was sexually abused by her counselor with outrage. You may want revenge; to prosecute the counselor so he never practices again. However, just as in dealing with the original abuser, the survivor is the one who needs control in handling the situation. To recover from her therapist's betrayal, she needs to be empowered to take action and make decisions on her own behalf. You can support her emotionally, listen to her, get angry with her, help her to research and get information, but it is up to her to decide if (and how) she wants to confront the therapist—face-to-face, through his licensing board, in civil court or criminal court, or not at all. The survivor's decision will be based on many factors, including the counselor's professional affiliation and the part of the country you live in. Laws protecting clients from therapist and clergy abuse vary geographically and across disciplines. (The penalties for professional abuse should be strong and uniformly enforced. Each profession needs to police itself; to investigate, treat, and punish helping professionals who exploit clients. This is a place where a lot more political organizing has to be done.)

Two excellent handbooks on this subject have been published by the Task Force on Sexual Exploitation by Counselors and Therapists of the Minnesota Department of Corrections. (See the Resource section for ordering information.) *It's Never O.K.* provides practical guidelines for dealing with therapist abuse. It comes in two versions: one for professionals (attorneys, counselors, legislators, clergy); the other for victims, partners, and victim advocates. The book for survivors and partners defines therapist abuse, talks about the warning signs of sexual exploitation, goes over the range of feelings survivor-victims have, and talks about "the wheel of options" for confronting the counselor. It closes with guidelines for screening a new therapist and a "client's bill of rights." Although written specifically with Minnesota law in mind, this booklet is still an excellent way for a sexually abused survivor to begin exploring his or her options.

One of the worst results of therapist abuse is that it teaches survivors that it's not safe to get help. It's hard for survivors to trust again when they've been betrayed in their quest for help. The fact is, there are many excellent, trustworthy counselors with tremendous integrity and great skills. Hopefully, the survivor will eventually be willing to try again; to cautiously approach another counselor so she can get the quality help she needs and deserves.

INTIMACY AND
COMMUNICATION

"There's a part of me that wants to work this through with him, but I'm scared of being rejected and tossed around like a yo-yo."

"All relationships have their give-and-take, but this one's had a lot more give than take."

"What's a normal relationship any-way?"

Sometimes I feel a need to be exposed to what a "normal" relationship is like; to be able to sort out what sorts of difficulties we would encounter if neither of us came from a history of abuse.

This is a common wish because so many people have been abused as children. Few of us have healthy models to emulate. We do the best we can and wonder if other people struggle as much in their relationships as we do.

Unfortunately, there is no such thing as a "normal" union by which to gauge your relationship. By their nature, relationships are quirky and unique, based as they are on the individual personalities and unique needs of the people involved in them.

It's easy to fall into a pattern where you blame every problem in your relationship on the fact that one or both of you was abused. But the fact is that you and the survivor would be having conflicts, struggles, and rough places even if neither of you had been abused. Long-term relationships have struggles. All couples have to grapple with conflicting and shifting needs. Any two people who form a partnership are going to have to deal with differences in the way they communicate, cope with stress, and resolve conflicts; with varying levels of sexual interest, and differing needs for intimacy and independence. People who were never abused vie for control. They fight. They have moments when they feel estranged and hate each other. They have times when they are deeply in love and it all seems worth it. There are ups and downs, times of feeling close and times of feeling apart. Although being with a survivor (or being a survivor yourself) adds to the complexity and intensity of these problems, you wouldn't be free of them even if both of you had the happiest childhood in the world. There is no happily-ever-after.

If you want some reassurance about this, talk honestly to a couple you respect who've been together longer than you. Ask them to tell you what it's really been like. Ask about their struggles and conflicts and compromises. Then talk to another couple. Then another. You'll see that "normal" encompasses pain, hard work, excitement, boredom, disappointment, love, closeness, distance, and joy; and varies widely from couple to couple. Rather than compare yourselves to some imaginary ideal, I suggest that you both sit down and set your own goals about what you want out of your relationship. Measure your success by your ability to work toward those goals.

It seems that when our relationship is going well, she is secure enough to explore the past and then all hell breaks loose. Is there an end to this cycle?

Yes. As survivors move through the cycles of healing, they eventually stabilize; their explorations of the past become less explosive, less disruptive, and shorter in duration. Eventually, questions and feelings about the past lessen in frequency, magnitude, and importance. Disruptions from the survivor's past will become the exception, not the rule.

It may seem paradoxical, but that fact that things fall apart when they're secure makes perfect sense. When a survivor begins to relax, feel loved and cared about, and gains a sense of safety, she can let down some of her defenses and relinquish her constant need for self-protection. As she unwinds and heals in one area, her attention can go to the next level of pain she needs to face. When survival needs no longer take precedence, she has room to deal with the emotional issues that are interfering with her life.

You might be thinking, "Oh, great! I'd rather *not* be such a safe haven. I'm loving and kind and safe, and *this* is what I get?" While feeling frustrated is natural, remind yourself that the work the survivor's doing now will ultimately make her much more capable of intimacy than she is right now. Your love and caring and the security of your relationship are providing her with an opportunity for healing she desperately needs. In the long run, it holds the potential to bring you closer.

DISTANCING

Intimacy was established rather quickly in my relationship, but as we got closer, barriers were erected. Why is it that as more trust and caring develops, more distance is needed?

This dynamic is common, yet very confusing. You're in a new relationship. Everything is fine and developing well, but as you get closer, things start falling apart. Just at a time when your relationship should be deepening in love and commitment, the survivor starts pulling away, acting out, setting wildly fluctuating limits, and testing you right and left. You feel bewildered. What the hell is going on?

Often, survivors manage superficial relationships fairly easily; but as the level of trust and commitment grows, they panic and start pushing you away. There are several possible reasons for this. First, the survivor may finally feel safe enough with you to allow the abuse to surface. Second, he may be trying to protect you from the "evil" or "badness" he feels inside himself. He feels toxic on the inside; he doesn't want his shame and bad feelings to pollute you. Third, he may be acting out his basic survival needs: as a child he was abused by someone he loved and trusted; he learned that people who love you also hurt you; that families are unsafe, dangerous places. As he gets closer to making a commitment to you, he feels like he's entering a family again. He feels trapped and hemmed in, and needs to escape: being in a family, a deepening relationship, feelings of vulnerability, and someone saying "I love you" are clear signs of danger. If he doesn't protect himself, he's sure to be annihilated. He's already been abused by someone he loved and trusted; he can't tolerate that kind of betrayal again.

One partner, Abby, described the way this dynamic played out in her relationship:

> Periodically when we're close, he turns to me and says, "I'm not in love with you anymore," just kind of out of the blue. I get hurt and withdraw, and then we go on. I think I cross some sort of emotional line with him where I get too close and he becomes afraid of me. The message from him is, "Just back off. Get away from me."

Intimacy is terrifying for survivors. If you can step back and see things from his perspective, his actions won't seem so crazy. You'll see that there's a direct correlation between his need to distance and his feelings of closeness to you. Thinking about it this way can be oddly comforting. One partner explained:

> When I feel unloved and deprived, I remind myself that he wouldn't be going through this if we weren't getting close. His need to distance is a barometer of how close and intimate he was able to get to me. When I realize we're going through this because he loves me, it really helps.

When you're struggling with a survivor's need to distance, the most important thing is to go slowly, to build in a lot of "time-outs" where you regroup individually before going further as a couple. Expect the survivor to need distance, to test you. (He's basically saying, "Are you big enough to contain all of me? Will you leave when you find out who I really am?") Expect an opposing reaction every time you make a step toward greater intimacy. Respect his need to pull away. Instead of fighting it, try to move with it. Each time you respect his limits and give him space, he'll move closer to you.

Try to anticipate the rhythm of getting close and moving away, getting close and moving away. Learn to dance with it. Talk about what's happening between you. Sometimes if you recognize a dynamic, you go a long way toward learning to work with it. And sometimes, as Abby did, you'll have unexpected breakthroughs:

> We went to therapy and both tried to be as honest as we could. I finally saw the person I was in love with. I hadn't seen him in three years. He came out and I saw him. It was incredible. We were able to say we loved each other. It was a flash of reality.

The other thing to consider is that you may have some fears of your own about getting close. When the survivor is doing all the pulling away, acting out, and testing, you get to be the "healthy" partner who's ready and willing to be close if only the survivor weren't acting out. Be honest with yourself. If the survivor were ready and willing, would you be the one pulling away? Maybe he's expressing the fear and ambivalence for both of you.

Couples often rush into a commitment, but only part of them is really present. Their fears and uncertainties and unmet childhood needs are hiding in the wings. "Love at first sight" often means both partners think they're going to magically find the parent they never had. Instant intimacy is a way we cover up the real terror we feel about being close. By the time we get to be adults, all of us have been hurt. It's not easy for any of us to risk again.

Going slowly, small step by small step, can be good for both of you. If you're building a long-term relationship, the crucial thing is not the speed or intensity with which you're involved, but how strong a foundation you build. Don't make the speed of your commitment a test of the caring between you. Take your time and bring all of yourself with you. Openly acknowledge your fears—both his and yours. It's the only way to build real, lasting trust. It's the only way to establish a new experience of love for the survivor and for you— love as a force that empowers and frees, rather than crushes, the human spirit. (See "Scott's Story" on page 284 for an inspiring example of how one couple creatively dealt with distancing.)

Why are survivors so rigid and inflexible?

Survivors don't have the corner on inflexibility. When we're scared of being hurt, we all have a tendency to get rigid. Inflexibility comes from fear. Flexibility requires a sense of trust that things will work out, that we can make mistakes, and that nothing terrible will happen as a result. Flexible people are creative thinkers; they see more than one solution to a problem. They feel confident dealing with situations moment by moment. They have no feeling of impending doom; they're free to shift their responses as a given situation changes because they don't feel like it's a matter of life and death.

Being flexible takes practice. Children learn about flexibility by growing up in an environment in which they can safely explore possibilities, make mistakes, experiment with different options, and shift course midstream. In abusive households, doing any of these things (in fact, doing anything but one narrow band of behavior) often has severe consequences including physical violence, material deprivation, and emotional or sexual abuse.

Being rigid is a poor attempt at creating safety; in fact it is less safe. Rigid people are so busy maintaining their boundaries and enforcing their own set of rules that they stop paying attention to what's really happening around them. They don't have the flexibility to change their response as a situation changes. They narrow their experience of life and can't bend to accomodate new information.

Rigid people think in terms of black and white: People are good or bad. You're a hero or you're a betrayer. You fail or you succeed. There is no room for the gray, for gradations. When we're locked into this kind of thinking, we end up feeling betrayed a lot. The betrayals are always betrayals with a "big *B*" because there is no room for mistakes, no margin of error. This holds true in the way we judge ourselves as well as the way we judge others.

Being rigid is also a way to fend off feelings: if there are no chinks in your armor, you don't have to feel. If you control your environment thoroughly enough, nothing unexpected will ever happen to you again. You know how you're going to respond to every situation; you don't have to be present in the moment, using your feelings to assess what's going on.

RIGIDITY

In big storms, it's the trees that bend with the wind that survive. Rigid structures are the ones that crumble.

Healing involves a dismantling of the rigid structures which protected us in childhood, but which limit our existence today. Giving up the structures is terrifying because there is tremendous vulnerability underneath. But as we heal our early pain, one of the by-products is an increase in our capacity for flexibility.

How can we gain control over the exaggerated need for control?

Control is a ruling force in many relationships. Survivors are not alone in having strong needs for control. Anyone raised in an environment that was out of control or dangerous grows up with a strong need for control. There is a power struggle in many relationships, and partners and survivors are no exception. One partner explained: "I need control. She needs control. So we butt heads a lot."

With passive survivors, it's sometimes the partner who wields the most control. That was true for Virginia (for more of her story, see page 293):

> I tried very hard to control Keith. How did I do it? I undermined his sense of confidence. Because of all the abuse in his childhood, he didn't start out with much self-confidence. I had kids before we got together; my subliminal message to him was, "I don't think you can do this right with the kids. I don't trust you." I wanted him to do everything my way. I didn't trust him to have his own instincts and feelings; to find things his own way. That really hindered him in terms of growing up, maturing, and being able to take responsibility. At the same time I was yelling at him to take responsibility for the kids, I was enclosing him in a net where he could only move an inch here and an inch there. That was really unfortunate. He's confronted me on that a lot.

No matter which one of you has more control in your relationship, the important thing is that change can occur. One man described the way his wife was gradually relinquishing her need for control in their relationship:

> Control? At the beginning, it was total. Now it's not so total. It's changed slowly over time. With what the kids wear. The kids used to have to look perfect. Now they can pick out their own clothes. With our house. Our house used to be the shame pit. If people came over and saw the

way we lived, it would never measure up to the way her mother kept house. Now she's able to say, "This is our house. If you don't like it, that's your business." In our daily interactions, I don't feel manipulated anymore. The control she tried to hold over my thoughts and feelings is almost gone. Control just isn't the issue it once was. The only area that hasn't changed is sex. She still needs total control over the initiation of sex. It doesn't work any other way. Yet. I hope it will. [For more on survivors' needs to control sex, see page 180 and 182]

Even though healing is a process of taking risks and becoming more flexible, it requires that the survivor have enough control to feel safe. To some extent, the partner with lesser needs for control has to put up with this. (And yes, complaining and negotiation are allowed.) If both of you have strong control needs, learn to take turns. As you trust each other more, the give-and-take in your relationship will reach a place of greater balance.

How can I convey the fact that I am worthy of trust?

Be trustworthy. Be reliable. Follow up and do the things you say you're going to do. Pay attention to details. Build a track record of being reliable. You build trust by being worthy of it.

Know your own limits. When you push yourself to give more (or promise more) than you're capable of, you invariably end up disappointing the survivor. She translates that into a belief that she can't trust you. If you set clear boundaries and tell the survivor what you can and can't be "trusted" to do, her expectations will be more in line with reality.

Don't expect the survivor to trust you automatically. Let her distrust exist in the relationship with you. It's part of what she comes with. Gradually, as you demonstrate that you can be trusted, her distrust will lessen and belief in you will take its place.

Remind yourself about what she's been through. When you think about her history, it makes sense that she has trouble trusting you. It's amazing that she trusts at all.

Children are born trusting. They have no reason *not* to trust. Ideally, young children experience themselves at the center of a universe full of loving, benevolent beings who watch out for them and tend to their needs. Their trust in their caretakers is absolute. In a nonabusive family, this trust is usually met with love, caring, and tenderness.

Children know nothing about deception, pain, and abuse until they are abused and lied to. They don't give up their trust easily; trust has to be beaten out of them through repetitive betrayals. This is what happened to the survivor: in the most painful way imaginable, her sense of trust was destroyed by the abuser.

The fact that the survivor loves you makes it no easier for her to trust you. Sometimes, in fact, it is more difficult for survivors to trust someone they love; their previous life experience has shown them that people who love them twist that love into hurt and betrayal. The survivor has had little or no experience to the contrary. Not yet. That's where you come in.

Unfortunately, you can't just say, "Trust me. You can trust me," and expect the survivor to abandon her protective defenses and bare her soft underbelly to you. Trust has to be built through shared experience, one small step at a time. As you come through for the survivor, again and again, she will slowly grow to trust you. Not because you told her she could trust you or because you know you're trustworthy or because you've been trustworthy with someone else, but because her concrete day-to-day experiences with you become strong enough to contradict the life experiences she's had until now. Be patient. (But if your feelings are hurt because she keeps telling you how untrustworthy you are, say so.)

Talk about what it would take for the survivor to trust you. She may expect some kind of superhuman perfection: you should always be sensitive, unwaveringly supportive, never late, constantly vigilant, and basically infallible. (Sounds kind of like the Boy Scouts, doesn't it?) That's unrealistic. No one is one hundred percent trustworthy. She isn't. (Doesn't she make promises and then break them because she had a memory and felt too overwhelmed to follow through?) You don't have to be, either. Perfection is not the basis for trust. Accountability is.

Define together what it means to be trustworthy. There may be areas in which you can be trusted absolutely (things that have to do with abuse, for instance), and others in which you're liable to make mistakes. Tell her, "You can trust me never to force myself on you sexually, but there may be times I'm late." Develop realistic expectations that allow for human fallibility.

Ultimately, trust is an act of faith, because none of us is perfect; none of knows the future. No matter how clear or solid our intentions are, we never know what events will happen that may deter us from those intentions. There is a calculated risk in every act of trust.

How do I get the survivor to keep agreements, negotiate in good faith, and not keep changing the ground rules?

This partner is expressing frustration at the tendency survivors have toward inconsistency. They say one thing, then change their minds. They say, "Yes, you can touch me here." Then they say, "No you can't." They say, "I want you to ask me how my therapy went," and then accuse you of prying when you ask. "But you told me to ask!" you counter. To no avail. You've violated the survivor's boundaries—again.

What's happening here is that the survivor is learning to set limits, something he's never done before. The learning process for limit-setting is trial and error—set a boundary, see how it feels, change it, see how it feels again. The survivor makes a promise, then realizes he's promised more than he can deliver, and doesn't come through. (This is something we all do at times.) He comes up with an elaborate plan for sexual contact between you, then backs off when he realizes he can't handle it. Why? Because he went to bed as a grown man, and turned into a frightened six-year-old when you touched him. His needs changed and he had to change with them. To keep a promise when he doesn't want to means he's doing something against his will. To him, this feels like the abuse.

If the survivor is near the beginning of his healing, you're dealing with someone for whom free choice has become a life-and-death issue. That translates for you into an awful lot of inconsistency. You can't trust him to follow through on anything. This can be exasperating. You want to be respectful of his limits, but his limits vary from one day to the next, sometimes from one hour or minute to the next. You're never on solid ground. The rules are always changing and he's the one with the rule book. This can be extremely frustrating.

The survivor's need for absolute control will diminish with time. Knowing that, however, doesn't necessarily make things easier for you right now. If you're feeling angry and frustrated, say so. The survivor may be so pleased to be taking care of himself (saying no) that he's not thinking about the effect his actions are having. Tell him. Let him know you're upset. Tell him why. If you're reaching your limit on "anything goes," say so.

One of the keys in working with a survivor who can't keep agreements is to start small. Survivors frequently promise more than they're capable of because they're afraid of displeasing or losing you. If you make it clear that you'd rather have him keep an agreement about a small thing than promise you the world, his agreements will stand a greater chance of holding firm. Instead of trying to have sex (and failing), maybe he can agree to talk about it for twenty minutes once a week (as long as he gets to choose the time). Agreeing to do something with an open-ended time frame gives the survivor more of a sense of control. Instead of feeling a sense of impending doom ("Now I have to . . ."), the survivor gets to decide in the moment when it's possible for him to follow through.

Right now, you're not dealing with someone whose resources and stability equal yours. But that doesn't mean there's not a small place where he can begin to respond consistently. See if you can set that as a goal between you. Then find a realistic place to begin.

My partner goes to a one-hour therapy session. I'm working fourteen hours a day. I'm tired. She cannot stop talking about incest. How can I peacefully stop her?

You and the survivor are experiencing conflicting needs. You need peace and a lack of stress at home. You're tired. Your back hurts. You've put in a long day. You want to kick back and watch TV. You're just starting to relax when the survivor comes in and starts telling you about the time she was five and her uncle put his fingers in her vagina. You want to listen. You want to be supportive. But what you're really dying to know is if the Celtics are ahead at halftime.

It's true that survivors need to talk. After years of silence, they've found their voices. That's fine with you. In fact, it's terrific. You support her in finding her voice. You just don't always want to be the one to hear it.

When I first remembered my abuse, I literally didn't talk about anything else for eighteen months. A year and a half after my first memories, I was having dinner with my friend Karen at Cha Cha Cha's, a Caribbean restaurant on Haight Street in San Francisco. After we finished our plantains, andouille sausage, black beans, and rice, had polished off the shrimp with garlic sauce, and were noisily munching on the Tootsie Rolls they serve with the check, she turned to me and said in amazement, "Laura, do you realize we just got all the way through dinner and you never once talked about sexual abuse?" I looked at her and smiled. I was stunned myself. I'd talked about sexual abuse for so long I couldn't remember ever not talking about it. It was over those Tootsie Rolls that I realized, for the first time, that the rest of my life might not be spent obsessing about being an incest survivor.

It's true that survivors need to talk. But you don't always have to be the one to listen. One of the most important tasks survivors face is to build a support system: a varied array of people who can listen, receive calls in the middle of the night, talk for hours, and care. Although you're an essential part of the survivor's support system, you are only one part, not the whole.

You need to set limits on how much (or when) you're willing to talk about sexual abuse. It's important that you be involved, that you take the time to listen and to care, but if you go beyond your own limits you'll find yourself glazed over, feigning attention, and eventually, resentful. That won't help either of you. In my experience, no one can listen to a survivor as much as she needs to talk except another survivor. It's okay to say no sometimes.

It's even okay to say no most of the time. If you're trying to break out of a pattern of caretaking, it's okay to ask the survivor to get her primary support elsewhere. If both of you are healing, there may be periods when you just can't listen to each other. That was true for Virginia and Keith:

> I didn't want to hear about his flashbacks, his therapy, or his ISA group.[1] For awhile he was calling me at work all the time, and I didn't want to be interrupted like that. I asked him to stop telling me. I didn't want to caretake him. I wanted him to bring his incest issues to his therapist, not to me. We made an agreement. If he wanted to tell me something, he could ask me and I would say "yes" or "no." But generally, when he had a flashback, or was panicked or fearful, I didn't want to hear it. He called someone else. He couldn't bear to hear about my pain or recovery either. When he tried to listen, he couldn't stay with my pain: he either got angry or switched it over to his pain. That always made me feel worse. And I couldn't resist analyzing him and his problems. So for a while, talking about any kind of deep issue was off-limits. We agreed to take those things to our therapists or to support group members, but not to each other. After keeping things separate for a while, we started to feel estranged. Now we're trying to come back to each other just a bit. I'm willing to listen a little more. So is he. But that's after a year of couples' therapy and a lot of individual work on both our parts. [For more of Virginia's story, see page 293.]

Think about what you need. What are you willing to give freely and without resentment? Can you listen an hour a day? Two nights

---

[1] Incest Survivors Anonymous, ISA is a 12-step fellowship for incest survivors. See the resource section for more information.

a week? Do you need Tuesdays off from talking about sexual abuse? Thursday nights as a time you go out and do something fun together, without talking about abuse? Your limits shouldn't be rigid, but they should provide you with a sense of protection that you're not on call twenty-four hours a day. (You will have to make exceptions for emergencies. That's something the two of you will have to work out ahead of time. You'll have to define for yourselves what constitutes an emergency. See page 84 for one method you can use.)

Wait until a time when the survivor isn't in a crisis (I know, sometimes that's difficult) to talk about what you need. Be gentle in your presentation. Reassure her that you support her and want to be there for her. Remind her that there's a difference between abandonment and healthy boundaries. Then choose your words carefully. Instead of saying, "I can't stand hearing this anymore. Leave me alone!" try saying, "If you want me to be there for you, I need some time to recharge. Here's what I propose . . ." Then state your idea. Ask, "How is that for you? Do you have any other suggestions?" Give yourself room to negotiate, but don't cave in. You deserve time and space that's free from listening to stories of sexual abuse.

Every scrap of advice to partners (and there are just scraps now) starts off by saying, "You have to listen to the survivor." This is very frustrating! My boyfriend won't talk to me! There's a barrier in the relationship. I'm working "blind." What can I do?

Communication is crucial to any working relationship. Yet it often becomes a critical problem between survivors and partners. Sometimes the survivor wants to talk too much, and you have to set limits to take care of yourself. Other times survivors are secretive about what they're doing in therapy, the steps they're taking to heal, resentful of any questions you ask. "I'm not ready to talk about it," they say. "I don't think you can handle it." All you have to work with is general information ("I was abused as a child and I'm looking into it"). But abuse does not affect your life in a general way. Your life is being turned upside-down, and on top of everything else that's going on, the survivor is shutting you out.

Survivors withhold information for a number of reasons. As a child, the survivor most likely suffered alone. His pain was hidden and private; he's not used to sharing it. For a lifetime, he may have kept the abuse a secret, perhaps even under threat of death. Secrecy becomes an ingrained pattern, difficult, and often terrifying to break. Yet silence gives the abuse more power and creates emotional distance between you, just when he needs your support the most.

The survivor may feel that the abuse is too painful to talk about. He's afraid it will hurt or shock you. Perhaps he worries that you'll minimize the damage and tell him to "get over it." (Even the most sensitive partners want to say this at times.) If the abuse has been hidden for some time, he's scared you'll say, "Why didn't you tell me before?" He's afraid of the way you'll react when you realize the problems you've been repeatedly blamed for really stem from the abuse. These are real fears on his part. You *will* react. You will not just be a smooth mirror beaming back support.

Another impediment to communication is the self-centered stage many survivors go through. (See "Self-absorption" on page 36.) Remind him that the abuse is affecting you too, and that if he wants your support, he has to be willing to involve you in his day-to-day struggles.

Although it can be scary for the survivor to talk about what he's going through, he needs to include you in his healing process. He doesn't have to tell you every detail (and you probably wouldn't want to hear them all), but you should have enough information to be an active participant.

If the survivor is reluctant or scared to talk to you, explore the reasons he's holding back. If they're connected to your behavior (you're hotheaded and are likely to rush out and confront the abuser) or your attitudes (you think dwelling in the past is a waste of time), you'll have to work on your receptivity before it will be safe for the survivor to talk to you. If the survivor's afraid of your anger, you may need a third person to facilitate your initial conversations. And if the problem is a fear of breaking silence, the survivor needs more support for breaking through the layers of secrecy.

Your life is being dramatically influenced by the survivor's choice to work on sexual abuse issues. You need and deserve information about what he's going through. Communication is not optional; it's a necessary risk the survivor has to take if he wants your support. The survivor may not feel comfortable overnight, and the opening up process may be slow, but over time he needs to learn to share his pain and struggles with you.

Being the partner of a survivor has become an important aspect of my life, but it feels like I shouldn't identify myself as such to others because it inadvertantly identifies my lover as a survivor. He's much more private than I am. What should I do?

Privacy is a tricky issue for many couples. Often, members of a couple have widely varying standards of what can be shared, and with whom. Some of us were raised in families with a "no talk" rule: "What goes on in this house stays in this house." Others were taught to freely discuss our problems in a community of extended family and friends. These two communication styles (and many in between) can lead to conflict. It's easy to form judgments about how your partner handles information: "He tells everyone everything." "She pretends everything is fine all the time." It takes time, respect for your partner's position, negotiation, and compromise to work out a family agreement on what gets talked about, when, and with whom.

When you're involved with a survivor, the issue of privacy gets even trickier. The survivor may not want you to tell people he's a survivor because he's ashamed, isn't ready for the information to get back to his family, or is afraid people will treat him differently (and in some cases, he may be right). He may want to talk for himself or he may not be ready to talk at all. Revealing personal information at his own pace provides him with a necessary sense of safety and control. On the other hand (and just as important), you need a safe place to talk about your feelings and experiences as a partner. Your life is being shaken up. You need sympathetic ears, encouragement, and help figuring out what to do. It's not fair for the survivor to limit your communication in such a way that it isolates you and leaves you without support.

What I say to survivors is this: "Your partner needs at least one person (and hopefully more) that he or she can freely confide in. You can have some say in the decision of who that person (or people) is, but it's not fair for you to say, 'I don't want you talking about this.' This is a place where you have to give, at least a little. If you want the support of your partner, you have to allow your partner to get support as well."

One man explained the way talking to friends works in his family:

She has rules about who I can talk to. It isn't rigid. If I need to talk about it with somebody to take care of myself, that's okay. But it has to be someone who can be trusted with the information, not just to chat about it.

Another partner, Virginia, described the way she works it out with her husband:

I've always had to have deep, personal friends that I can talk to, even about the most intimate problems with Keith. There are only one or two that know everything, but I couldn't do it without them. Keith gets nervous about me talking to other people. He gets scared. Sometimes he tells me, "Don't tell so-and-so." And often I'll ask his permission if I need to talk about something. But sometimes I don't. If I'm really in crisis, I just go and talk to one of those really close people. If I need to talk that badly, I do it anyway. Afterwards, I tell him. He may be a little blown away, but he always says it's okay. It's hard for him to know that other people know the details of what happened to him. He knows the people I've told, and it's been painful for him at times. He still feels ashamed. But my whole life was secrets and I can't keep them anymore. I think I keep them appropriately. This is not something I spread around the universe, but I can't keep it all inside my own head either. I need more of an outlet than just an hour a week with a therapist. I need to talk things out with my friends; afterwards I feel much better. Keith knows that. It's not easy for him, but on the whole he's been very supportive. [For more of Virginia's story, see page 293.]

When choosing someone to talk to, try to find someone who cares about the survivor as well as you. At a minimum, they should have an open mind about the survivor's process. That way, you'll get support for your feelings and needs without being drawn into a character assassination of the survivor. Being assured that you know the difference between "talking about feelings" and "trashing him" will help to set the survivor's mind at ease.

If the survivor is afraid about you talking to a particular person, ask why. Is it because the person you want to tell is close to his uncle?

Won't handle the information respectfully? Has a reputation for gossiping? Maybe you have chosen the wrong person. Or maybe there's a way to structure the interaction that will make the situation feel safer for the survivor. Working out ground rules ahead of time can help to allay some of his fears: "I'll ask Roger not to tell anyone else and explain why it's important." "I'll join a partners' group and only talk intimately to the people I meet there."

Sometimes, though, regardless of how many ground rules you set, the survivor still feels scared and doesn't want you to say anything. In that case, talk anyway. Choose the person carefully, but go ahead and talk. Your emotional well-being and ability to stay in the relationship depend on it.

One place where you will have to respect the survivor's wishes fully is around his family. It's critical that the survivor have control over when, if, and how he talks to his family about the abuse. (For more on dealing with the survivor's family, turn to page 211.) But outside the realm of his family, you have a right to find safe people you can confide in.

How do I deal with her feeling like she's "bad" every time I become critical or angry or irritated about something?

What the survivor is doing is personalizing every conflict. She's unable to separate her actions and behaviors from who she is as a person. She doesn't see the difference between criticism of her behavior and criticism of her as a person. Her self-esteem is not yet strong enough for her to hold her own in a conflict: she caves in and assumes she is "bad." Any criticism reinforces her poor self-image.

It's likely that in her family growing up, criticisms and feedback weren't geared to change behavior but to annihilate character. Instead of being told to do her homework, she may have been told, "You're stupid." Instead of being asked to do the dishes, she heard, "You're lazy. You'll never amount to anything." This kind of steady character assassination in childhood annihilates a child's sense of self and leads to terrible problems with self-esteem later on. The child stops defending herself and takes every criticism as an accurate assessment of her "rotten" character. She feels responsible for everyone else's feelings and blames herself for the abuse.

As an adult, this leaves the survivor feeling self-hating and insecure. She blames herself for everything and presents a fragile self to the world. She isn't capable of handling the natural conflicts and feelings that arise in a relationship: every time you have a conflict, she falls apart. Your energy shifts from addressing your concern to helping her out of the bottomless pit she's fallen into. Instead of being able to creatively solve the original problem, you end up taking care of her. The focus shifts to her needs, and yours are left far behind. You feel angry, left out, and resentful.

The survivor may not be consciously trying to control you, but that's what's happening: your feelings and needs are being contained and controlled. You learn that any discussion of your needs leads her to collapse and bury herself in self-hatred. You don't want to upset her or to make her feel worse about herself than she already does, so you start tiptoeing around her.

This is a mistake. If you always protect her from the inevitable stresses of real life, you help maintain her sense of frailty. She needs to learn to handle conflict without falling apart. (This doesn't give you license to overwhelm her with your anger; you can learn to be honest *and* sensitive.)

Basically, what you're dealing with is a self-esteem problem. The survivor needs to build up enough of a sense of self that she can stand up to you, fight back, and discuss problems in your relationship without having her basic core self threatened. As she heals, her self-esteem will naturally increase; you should see a steady improvement.

In the meantime, there are several things you can do. Be conscious of the way you express criticism. Instead of making judgments ("You're selfish/demanding/difficult"), talk about specific problem behaviors and how they affect you. Give the survivor lots of reinforcement about her core self: tell her you think she's a great and lovable person; you just don't like this particular thing she's doing. Also, try a more structured approach to talking (see page 169 for some ideas) or seek out the help of a couples' counselor. This can be a tough issue to negotiate on your own.

Finally, take care of yourself. If you're sick of being careful and need to be your loud, boisterous, sometimes tactless self, tell the survivor, "That's it. I need a break." Spend some time with people who are thick-skinned; who don't care what you do or say. Don't be careful. Stop stifling yourself. Be your imperfect self, as fully and naturally as you can.

My wife feels threatened by issues on which we don't agree. Whenever I state my needs, she says I'm trying to control her. How can we resolve this?

Conflicting needs are normal in a relationship. No matter how scary it is for the survivor, you need room to have feelings and needs that differ from hers. There's nothing wrong with disagreements, although they require compromise, some old-fashioned give-and-take.

You both need to learn the difference between stating a need and making a demand: demands are nonnegotiable; there's a price to pay if the giver doesn't comply. Stating a need is different: it shouldn't have a price tag attached. When you say "I want" or "I need," you are expressing a wish or a desire. The other person should have flexibility in the way they respond. When you state your needs, there should be room for the other person to say yes or no; to negotiate a compromise.

Talk to the survivor about what makes your needs so threatening. Is it the way you communicate your needs that frightens her? Is she afraid you'll leave if you don't get your way? Does she feel obliged to sacrifice her needs to meet yours (like she did with the abuser)? What happened in her childhood home when there was a disagreement? Did it spell disaster?

Maybe the survivor has never experienced or participated in a successful negotiation. Her only experience might be that when someone wanted something from her, she lost herself and got hurt every time. That's a strong motivation for avoiding conflict.

In order for the survivor to relax and allow more differences between you, she's going to have to gradually build up a new base of experience. You can begin by coming up with ground rules for negotiating. They will create a framework within which it feels safer to disagree. (Turn the page for detailed suggestions on how to do this.)

Be creative. If the survivor feels terribly threatened when you disagree face-to-face, try writing her a letter instead. Or take turns: each of you gets five uninterrupted minutes to say whatever it is you're feeling before the other person can respond. Practice active listening. (See page 70 for an example.) Save your most difficult talks for couples' counseling.

FEAR OF CONFLICT

Ultimately, the survivor needs to experience that you can disagree (or even have a fight) and be close again afterwards. She'll have to see that you can live through her saying no, and that she can do the same. These changes are slow and take time, but positive experiences with you ease her deep-seated fears.

Whenever my lover and I try to talk about the things we want from each other, we end up in a power struggle. He says I have to do things his way because he's a survivor. I say that's not fair, that my needs count too. We end up in a stalemate, both feeling angry, let down, and discouraged. What can we do?

Learning to negotiate conflicting needs is one of the cornerstones of a successful relationship. Without respectful negotiation, it's easy to get lost in competition and resentment. Yet few of us have had the opportunity to learn about successful negotiation. Many of us grew up in families where the biggest, strongest, loudest (or sometimes, most vulnerable) person got what he or she wanted. We learned that life was about competing for limited resources; that each interaction held a winner and a loser. Certain behaviors, we found, helped us win more frequently; we still use many of them with great regularity. They include (but are not limited to): bullying, threatening, whining, complaining, manipulating, withholding, and acting like a victim.

Cooperative problem-solving begins with a different set of assumptions: Everyone's needs and feelings are important. There isn't a shortage of resources. More than one person can win at a time. Everyone gets some of what he wants. Compromise is not the same as losing.

To negotiate successfully, you have to develop an attitude of respect for the other person's feelings and point of view. Being respectful doesn't mean you have to give the other person everything he wants: you'll still have differences, but you'll both feel cared about and listened to. You should come away from a successful negotiation feeling like allies: "I'm getting some of what I want; so is he." "He's willing to stretch for me. I'm willing to challenge myself for him too." "If he could give it to me, he would."

Successful negotiation isn't easy. Any time someone says "I want" or "I need," the discussion frequently disintegrates into a power struggle where both partners pull out all their old manipulative and defensive tricks. The guidelines which follow provide an alternative; they establish a safe structure for discussing conflicting needs. Many couples have used these guidelines to resolve long-standing barriers to communication.

LEARNING TO NEGOTIATE

If you haven't already done so, complete a list of your needs and wants according to the instructions on page 75. When you're through, take each want or need you marked "partner" or "partner only" and translate it into something concrete you can ask for: "I don't want to talk about sexual abuse on Tuesday and Thursday nights." "I want you to listen to me for at least a half hour a week while I talk about my problems."

As you compile your list, be realistic. Ask for gradual movement over time rather than instant change. If the survivor can't bear to be touched because he's bombarded with flashbacks every time you touch him, asking for ecstatic sex isn't very realistic. Try "I want to steadily and slowly rebuild our sexual life together. I need you to tell me that you want this too."

You'll have more chance of success if you ask for something that gives the survivor some room ("I need to reestablish some kind of sexual expression between us") rather than being so specific that there's no flexibility or give ("We have to start having sex again"). The more space you leave to negotiate a mutually workable solution, the more likely you are to get what you want.

State each need as a positive statement of action. Don't hide a criticism or a barb in your statement. Instead of saying, "I want you to stop being such a jerk when you get angry," say, "I need you to find more constructive ways to express your anger."

The examples below are to get you started. Feel free to copy down any that apply to you. Add as many others as you can think of.

I want you to talk to me when you feel like withdrawing.

I don't want to eat dinner with your brother unless I can freely speak my mind.

I don't want your parents babysitting anymore.

I want you to acknowledge how hard this is for me.

I want to reestablish some kind of physical relationship with you.

It's okay for me to hurt. I want you to listen and acknowledge that my pain is important too.

I want you to find some small way to nurture me on a regular basis.

I want you to reassure me that you want our sex life to get easier too.

I want to have fun with you at least once a week.

I want you to go to couples' counseling with me.

I want to be able to talk honestly to at least one other person about the details of what's going on in our relationship.

I want to be able to take time off without recriminations.

I want credit and appreciation for what I'm doing.

When you're done, look back over your list. Put a check mark next to anything that is absolute, a core thing you must have to continue in your relationship. These are your bottom lines, things that are not open to compromise or negotiation. Bottom lines draw a fixed boundary and should only be used in extreme situations: "I don't want your parents babysitting anymore." "I want you to make a commitment not to kill yourself." "I want you to agree not to have any more affairs."

Choose your bottom lines carefully; they shouldn't be used to manipulate or force your partner into giving you what you want. They should genuinely reflect your true limits. If your partner can't say yes to your bottom lines, that's an indicator that you may need to leave the relationship. (For more on leaving or staying, see page 87.)

Most things on your list should be open to negotiation. ("I want us to go to couples' counseling" might change to "I want us to actively set aside time to talk about our problems.") They represent things you need over time; changes you'd like to work toward. These might be modified by finding a smaller, more manageable step you could both agree to.

Separately from you, the survivor should make a comparable list. Don't share your lists until you've both finished. If you share prematurely, you'll have more of a tendency to censor or tone down what you ask for. (But feel free to add new things to your list at any time, even if you're stealing ideas from your partner.)

Your respective lists will give you a good starting point for negotiating necessary changes in your relationship. When you come back together to share what you've written, it will be immediately apparent where your needs dovetail and where they're incompatible. You will see the places you can easily work together and the ones where you're stuck.

You may be able to talk through some of the easier areas yourselves, but need to hold off on discussing the more volatile ones until you can meet with a third person. Enlist the help of a counselor to serve as a witness/mediator. If you're scared, haven't been able to discuss your situation honestly before, or are heading into territory that is threatening for either of you, a few sessions with a couples' counselor can help your communication enormously.

If you decide to talk on your own, choose a time when you won't be disturbed and when there isn't already a lot of tension between you. Remind each other that the purpose of this conversation is to allow each of you to get more of what you need, to create more balance in your relationship, and ultimately, to make you closer. Take a few minutes to discuss your fears before you begin.

Start by setting ground rules for your conversation. Ground rules are limits you both agree to before you start to talk. They create more of a feeling of safety between you: your conversation is contained; you agree that certain lines won't be crossed. Here are some sample ground rules:

- If this degenerates into a fight, we'll stop.
- If either of us feels like we're digging ourselves into a deeper hole, we'll make an appointment with a counselor to help us.
- Let's remind each other to breathe.
- Humor is appreciated, as long as we don't laugh at each other.
- Either of us can call a time-out or ask for reassurance at any time.
- We'll talk for two hours and then we'll do something easy and relaxed for the rest of the afternoon.
- We won't criticize each other for having needs we can't meet.

Write down your ground rules before you start talking. Then read your lists to each other. You can take turns, item by item, or read your entire lists in turn. Make it clear which things (if any) are bottom lines.

As much as you can, listen with an open mind, instead of judging, "That's ridiculous! I can't believe you're asking for that!" or immediately reacting from a place of fear, "Oh my God! He wants me to do *that*?" If you feel confused or need clarification, ask questions. Your first job is to clearly understand what your partner is asking for. You'll get to respond later.

After you've gone through your lists the first time, go back and discuss each item. In some cases, your needs will be complementary. Other times they will be in direct opposition. Some will fall in the middle. It's generally easier to start with those items that are easier and less emotionally charged, and work up to the harder ones. You may want to put the hardest topics aside until you can meet with a counselor.

For each item, discuss what is or isn't realistic in meeting that goal. It's better to succeed at a smaller, more manageable task than to fail at fulfilling an unrealistic promise. Try to be honest with yourself. What could you actually do in the next two weeks? In the next month? In the next six months? If your partner has needs you'd like to meet, but you don't feel capable right now, see if there's a smaller step you can begin with.

For each item you can agree to, come up with an action plan. What will you do? What will your partner do? On a separate piece of paper, write a short, concrete statement about the actions you agree to take. That way you'll be able to evaluate your progress later on. Sample statements are: "I will tell you I'm reaching my limits before I reach them." "I won't contact your family unless you want me to." These statements become personal goals for you. They represent your part of working together for change.

Here are some of the goals one partner came up with:

I'll investigate the possibility of joining a partners' group. If one doesn't exist, I'll take steps to start one.

I'll make a commitment to take a time-out before my anger explodes.

I'll make two social plans with friends on my own in the next month.

I'll be sensual and affectionate with John without coming on to him sexually afterwards.

The survivor came up with these:

I'll tell Sandy whenever I start to disappear emotionally.

Instead of shutting down sexually and withdrawing, I'll stay connected and talk about what I'm feeling.

I'll let Sandy go out with friends without crying and recriminations.

I'll look into joining a survivors' group.

When you've each come up with a list of goals, discuss means for assessing your progress. In two weeks, what should you have accomplished? In a month, how will you know if you've moved closer to your goals? How will you measure your progress? How will you know if your bottom lines are being met? What will you do if they're not?

Set a specific time to come back and look at your lists. Together, assess how you're each doing. Evaluate your progress without judgments or accusations. This is a trial-and-error process. If the survivor failed to do what he said he would, why did he fail? If you didn't follow through on your promises, what stood in your way? Try not to judge each other. Reaffirm your commitment to your goals, and talk about the things that got in your way. Are there modifications that need to be made? Set another time to check in on your progress. And don't forget to affirm the things that have worked. Celebrate any successes, no matter how small.

Will she love me in the end?

I wish I could answer that question with a definitive yes, but there are no guarantees. No one can look in a crystal ball and tell you that your relationship will work out if you stick it out.

Life is a gamble. Fifty percent of marriages end in divorce. The statistics are even worse for unmarried couples. You're going through a trying time right now, and either you'll make it or you won't. All you can control is your part—what you learn, how you love, what you do, how long you stay. The rest is up to her.

That's the problem with relationships: you can't control the outcome. Make the most of this moment, the time you have together now. There are no guarantees. (If you're the one thinking about leaving, see page 87.)

SEX

"It's like the abuser's hand is reaching out of the grave to fuck up my sex life. I hate it."

"I feel left out of the world of normal sexual functioning."

"I sometimes feel like a failure. If you're out there in the world competing for sexual partners and you pick one who's got a lot of problems, it means you didn't cut it on finding a lover."

"I masturbate a lot. It's a fact of life."

Why do we enjoy sexual relations less now than before therapy?

There's probably a lot more honesty in your sexual relationship than there was before. Many times survivors get by sexually by covering up their real feelings, dissociating (splitting off from themselves), hiding in fantasies, or going through the motions and faking it. It can be a shock (and a blow to your ego) to realize that your lover has only been pretending to enjoy making love with you. Or to find out that he's only climaxed because he imagined his father having sex with him. Or that he's physically enjoyed sex with you but was a million miles away emotionally. Once survivors begin to get in touch with what they are really feeling in their bodies, once they stop numbing out, they frequently get in touch with just how threatening and scary sex is for them.

Try not to take this personally. I hesitate writing that sentence, "Don't take it personally," because I know it's probably one of the most difficult pieces of advice for you to hear. "Don't take it personally? Don't take it *personally?!?* What could be more personal than finding out my lover hasn't been present when we've made love? What's more personal than being told he pretends I'm his father so he can climax? How much more personal can you get???"

Although the survivor's real feelings may feel like a terrible rejection of you, your body, and your sexuality, remember that the survivor is responding the way he is because of the abuse he suffered as a child. He was programmed to disconnect from sex, to disconnect from anyone who loved him and wanted to have sex with him. Although his feelings affect you personally, they probably don't have to do with anything you have or haven't done. They probably don't have to do with your skills as a lover or your value as a mate. They also are not a good indicator of the love the survivor has for you. He may love you very much; it's just that it's too scary to feel that in his body, too.

When the survivor starts being honest with you (and with himself), you may be shocked, angry, and bewildered, particularly if the two of you enjoyed sex before (or at least you thought you did). These are natural reactions. The experience you're having right now —having the sexual rug pulled out from under you—is very common. Sudden upheaval around sexual issues is the norm when survivors begin to work on abuse issues. Structures built on shaky ground have to be torn down before they can be rebuilt on a strong foundation.

Before I remembered the abuse, I had many lovers. I enjoyed sex with them. They enjoyed sex with me. But when I look back, I can see there was a way I wasn't connected. Because I didn't have any basis for comparison, I didn't know that everyone didn't space out and disappear during sex. I thought that was normal. I never found it odd that my sexual interest declined as my relationships got closer. I thought that was normal, too. If you'd asked me about my sex life, I would have told you that I was happy, that I was fine sexually. But that's because I wasn't really paying attention. I was doing it by rote. It was only when I started to delve into the abuse that my sex life fell apart. I'd try to do the sexual things that had worked for me for years, and to my chagrin, they didn't work anymore. I realized, in more ways than one, that I'd been living a lie, and I couldn't do it anymore. I had to go back and examine the damage. Only then could I begin the arduous process of rebuilding my sexual life from scratch.

For years after I started healing, I said to myself (and to anyone who cared to listen), "I wish I'd never opened up this can of worms. I'd rather be numb and unconscious. At least then I was enjoying myself." I would have given anything to shove the whole mess back into the closet. But I wouldn't say that now. For all the struggles I've had sexually, I'm glad I've woken up. Going through the motions, doing it because it's expected, is no longer acceptable to me. I respect myself more now. I have a deep need to take care of myself. Now that I know what it's like to really connect sexually and emotionally, I don't want to settle for less.

When a survivor takes in the fact that he's been sexually abused, he makes more room for the truth in his life. More of him comes alive. These new parts are often born in an atmosphere of pain and struggle, but as he moves through the pain, eventually, more of him becomes available. Ultimately, there will be more of him to love you. He will be able to make love intact—with the fullness of his passion, his vulnerability, his weaknesses, his strengths—not as an impostor. I know there will be times you'll wish the impostor had stayed around, but healing from childhood sexual abuse is a one-way trip.

There is no turning back. And the survivor has to bring all the undeveloped, hurt parts of his body, spirit, and mind with him. Be patient. At the other end will be a mature, intact adult, not a needy, wounded child. Isn't that who you really want to make love with?

My lover keeps saying she's not ready to deal with sex. I want to know when she will be. Where does sex fit in?

Unfortunately, sex is not usually something survivors can tackle at the beginning of the healing process. They're generally too preoccupied with flashbacks, panic attacks, self-destructive feelings, shame, terror, and survival to really pay attention to sex. In my experience, and in the experience of the hundreds of couples I've talked to, deep, lasting sexual healing is something that's only achieved in the later stages of healing.

When survivors try to tackle these issues because they're afraid their partners will leave and not because they're really ready, their efforts generally backfire. If you pressure the survivor to be sexual ("We have to make love or I'll leave." "We need to have sex twice a week"), that pressure feels like the original abuse and only shuts her down further. The survivor caves in and goes through the motions, adding on another layer of abuse to the abuse she's already experienced. But when you find a way to take the pressure off, you give her room to see that she actually does want to heal sexually, for her own reasons.

When I talk to survivors alone and ask them what they want sexually for themselves, and not for their partners, to maintain their relationships, or to make peace, they say things like: "I want to know what sex could be for me; what I would feel about sex if I hadn't been abused." "I'm curious. I don't know what it means, but I want my body back."

As a partner, you have a choice. You can leave your relationship and find someone else who will have sex (and enjoy sex) the way you want to. The survivor can't. If you separate and she gets in another relationship, she will find herself dealing with the same problems. Unless she heals sexually, she will be struggling with these issues for the rest of her life. In many ways, her motivation to change is greater than yours.

You cannot make someone heal sexually. You can't set the deadlines or orchestrate her progress. You can set mutual goals and work toward them. You can ask for the things you want, but you can't make her give them to you. You can say that sex is important to you and that you want, eventually, to have a mutual sexual relationship that is relaxed and feels good to both of you. Even if she can't give that to you now, the survivor should reach inside herself and find a way to tell you, "Yes, I want that, too. Over time, I want to reach a place where I feel good sexually, where I'm no longer haunted by my stepfather, where I can meet you deeply in a sexual way." If the survivor can at least give this to you, her wish to heal sexually, it gives you a chance to become aligned. (For more on establishing a common sexual goal, see pages 187 and 196.)

When I had my first memories of incest, seven years ago, my partner found herself in a relationship with someone who went from being very sexual, to being partially shut down, to being totally shut down. I had flashbacks every time she touched me, couldn't bear to be touched, changed my mind constantly: "Yes, I want sex." "No, I don't." After six months, she got fed up and left me. "I need to make love with my lover," she said. "I can't do this anymore."

My partner today has a very different experience. She finds herself involved with someone who enjoys being touched (most of the time), knows herself sexually, sets clear boundaries, likes to explore, and has an expansive view of sex. My partner has room to explore her own pockets of sexual pain. Sex is a place for us to connect, heal, express love, and have fun.

If you're involved with someone who can't make love at all, or who needs so much control that you feel shoved out entirely, it's hard to imagine that things can change sexually. But they can and do. Working with a survivor on sexual healing takes an incredible amount of patience, persistence, and an acceptance of the fact that you are growing, too. If you can find these things in yourself and stick it out over the long haul, things will change.

How long will my celibacy in marriage last?

In order to get in touch with their own sexuality, many survivors need to take a break from sexual pressure or expectations of any kind. A chosen period of celibacy may be necessary before they can begin the process of healing sexually. This time off may take a period of months or even longer. If you're already feeling sexually deprived, the idea of the survivor taking a vacation from sex may feel terrible to you, but you have to take into account the potential long-term gain. You can either keep struggling along as you are now, with no chance of change, only more alienation, or you can take the risk of letting go now, in the hope of real mutuality later on. Unless the survivor learns to say "no," her "yes" will never be meaningful.

A break from sex allows the survivor to focus on more critical aspects of her healing (recovering memories, dealing with the abuser, building a support system, believing the abuse took place). It is also a time to release some of the pressure that has built up between you. Instead of always wondering, "Are we going to make love?" "Is she going to reject me again?" you have clear boundaries to work with.

A break from sex is not a time to turn away from each other. In fact, many couples find they are so relieved to stop fighting about sex, they feel closer than they did before. They find creative ways to be intimate, and the survivor's trust grows ("My partner cares enough about me to take a break from sex"). This kind of trust is essential to the sexual rebuilding you will engage in later on.

I can't answer the question "How long?" Different survivors will need to take different amounts of time off. One survivor may need six weeks, another three months, and a third, a year or more. Once the survivor is ready to explore sexually again, she needs to go at her own pace (which will probably be excruciatingly slow for you). This can be easier to accept if you understand the way sexual abuse interferes with natural sexual development. The survivor stopped growing sexually at the time the abuse began. Her normal sexual evolution was cut short. She stopped experiencing pleasure in exploring her body and instead had to defend herself against adult sexuality, which was often mixed with violence and a confusing combination of pain, pleasure, and humiliation. She found a way to respond (or not respond) to the abuser, and left herself, and her own innocent sexual awakening, far behind. Her task now is to dig down under the layers of painful associations with sex and explore her innate sexual feelings, the ones that would have developed naturally if abuse hadn't gotten in the way.

To do this successfully, the survivor needs to slow way down and go back to the point when she stopped growing sexually. She needs to pace her involvement so she can start developing positive associations with sex. For a survivor who was abused in infancy, this might mean going back to the simple pleasure of movement and exploring space. For another survivor, flirting and holding hands may be the place she stopped developmentally. A third may need to act out the teenage rites of courtship and dating. (Not necessarily with other people; it can happen with you.) The thread running through all of these stages is that the survivor needs to have the control and needs to be able to say "no" and "stop" at any time. (And no, it doesn't take the survivor as many years to "grow up sexually" as it does in real life.)

As a partner, this means taking the back seat and letting the survivor control your sexual life for a time. "But she already controls it now!" you scream. "She says no and pushes me away all the time! You want me to give up the few crumbs I do get? I'm already feeling deprived. Why should I give up more?" It's absolutely natural to feel frustrated and angry, and to resist her need for more control, but if you let those feelings predominate, it will only make things harder for you. One partner explained: "It's easy for me to feel like a victim: 'Thirty-five years old and I still don't have a good sex life. Waaaaaaah!' It's pretty much a downward spiral from there."

As long as you stay in a power struggle over sex, you'll both be miserable. It's best to acknowledge and respect the survivor's need for a break from sex. When you choose to say "no" together, you begin to work as allies. What starts out feeling like deprivation can actually yield positive results for both of you. (See "Eric's Story" on page 265 for one couple's positive experience taking a break from sex.)

SEXUAL DESIRE

Is it unrealistic to expect that my girlfriend will ever increase her sexual desire? Can a person "learn" to desire sex?

People naturally have different levels of sexual desire. Some people want to have sex daily and others would be perfectly happy making love once every other month. Levels of sexual interest can be connected to sexual abuse, or they can just be a natural part of a person's personality, like a preference for rising early or staying up late. Even if your partner had never been sexually abused, it's quite possible she wouldn't want sex as much, or as infrequently, as you do.

There are many factors that can influence sexual desire: age, illness, disability, fatigue, weight gain or loss, childbirth and parenting, drug or alcohol use, stress, lack of sexual information, early rigid conditioning about sex ("sex is dirty," "sex is only for making babies," "just lay back and endure it"), lack of intimacy in a relationship, poor sexual technique, pressure to perform sexually, repressed anger, the turning of the seasons, or even a crummy haircut.

Sexual abuse is one of a myriad of factors that affects desire; it can obscure the survivor's natural interest in sex. Many survivors associate desire with a scary, out of control force—the desire of the abuser who used sex to hurt them. Sexual desire is not associated with love, tenderness, or pleasure. This includes your sexual desire. Many survivors wish their partners' desire for sex would just go away. One partner explained, "I've had to work to make her realize that my desiring sex is normal, healthy, and okay even though it creates difficulties for her and for us."

The survivor may see her own desire as a threatening force as well. When she's aroused sexually, she's afraid of becoming like the abuser. She doesn't want to abuse you (or herself), so she cuts off sensation instead.

There may also be dynamics in your relationship that are getting in the way of the survivor's desire. If you aren't getting enough (or any) sexual contact, and therefore are the one who always initiates sex, you may have to back off from being the initiator. As long as you are the one who wants and asks for sex, there is no room for the survivor to feel her own desire—she's too busy responding to (and sometimes, fending off) yours.

The survivor may also feel that any expression of desire on her part means that she will have to "go all the way." If she has never learned to say no or to stop sexual activity midstream, desire becomes a runaway train with only one possible destination. She fears that you will insist on sex if she expresses any sexual interest at all. She thinks, "If I feel desire, I have no choice but to go through with it." "Going through with it" involves some combination of gritting her teeth, pretending she isn't there, or counting cobwebs on the ceiling. That's what she did with the abuser, and it may be what she's doing with you. It's painful and she hates it. Therefore, she stops feeling desire as a way to protect herself.

Before a survivor can explore her own sexual desire, she needs to feel safe. Part of safety is knowing she can stop at any time, that your goal is connection and intimacy, not "going all the way." She also needs to know that you're both capable of handling the feelings that will invariably come up when she does allow herself to feel desire. If she starts feeling disgusted when she gets aroused, how will you handle it? If she suddenly gets sick to her stomach and has to throw up, what will you do? If she needs to say no to you again, right in the middle of making love, because she took the risk of starting, will you react angrily? She needs to know that you will be with her no matter what happens; that she won't be abandoned at a vulnerable moment. *She needs to know that you care more about her than you do about sex.* That's a trust that takes time to develop. As her positive associations with sex increase (that she doesn't have to "put out," that she can say no and not be abandoned, that small steps forward can feel good), her interest in being sexual will naturally increase.

As survivors uncover their own natural sexual impulses, they can experience more desire, less desire, or no significant change in their level of desire. Physical desire is not always reliable or consistent. However, physical desire is not necessary to make love. Interest alone is enough. This concept was pioneered by sex therapist JoAnn Loulan when she introduced the concept of sexual "willingness" in her breakthrough book, *Lesbian Sex*.[1] Willingness provides an alternative to traditional models of the sexual response cycle, in which sexual arousal always precedes sexual activity. Willingness can exist on an emotional or intellectual level; it doesn't have to be physical.

---

[1] JoAnn Loulan, *Lesbian Sex* (San Francisco: Spinsters/Aunt Lute, 1984).

SEXUAL DESIRE

Even if the survivor isn't having a single sexual sensation in her body, she can still say, "I'd like to explore sexually today. I want to go one step further. I'm willing to begin." Willingness is a way of saying yes, even if desire, in the traditional sense, isn't there. When a survivor knows that she can say yes simply because she is willing, the possibilities for exploring sexually are freed up tremendously.

How can I have a close, tender relationship with the survivor when flashbacks can occur so suddenly and be so disruptive?

Flashbacks refer to vivid remembrances of abuse. The survivor feels as if he's reexperiencing aspects of the original trauma. Flashbacks can be visual (seeing images), auditory (hearing conversations or other sounds), or kinesthetic (feeling body sensations). They can also involve taste and smell. One of the most common times for flashbacks to occur is during lovemaking. Survivors experiencing flashbacks can go numb, feel physical pain, nausea, arousal, terror, or disgust. Sometimes the survivor is aware of what is going on and can talk about it. Other times he seems to disappear. He may regress back to the age he was when the abuse took place, mix you up with the abuser (see page 95 for more), or otherwise confuse the past and the present. (For more on regression, see page 102.)

Flashbacks are disruptive and frightening. One minute you're making love with an adult, and the next you're with a sobbing eight-year-old. You feel as if the abuser has invaded your bed. (And you're right.) Something important is going on and you find yourself shut out. You don't know what to do, and you take it personally. But flashbacks aren't about you; they're about the body's need to tell its stories. Disturbing as they are, flashbacks are one of the primary ways survivors get information about their histories. You can't eliminate flashbacks because you don't want them to happen. Work at integrating flashbacks into your lovemaking instead.

Usually we approach sex with a set series of actions in mind. First you kiss, then you touch each other's bodies, take off your clothes (or leave some of them on), stimulate each other's genitals, have an orgasm (or orgasms), and fall asleep. When you make love with a survivor this all changes.

If you want to make love and be awake, be really alive and with the other person, you have to follow whatever it is that comes up between you. This could include incredible passion, moments of sadness, sobbing when someone has an orgasm (or because they can't), losing an erection, pictures of the survivor's father flashing in front of his eyes. Making love this way can bring up feelings for you, too. You might be fine one minute; the next, you're remembering your first sexual experience when you were young and scared and had to pretend you knew what you were doing. You never thought about it this way before, but suddenly you realize how terrified you were, how scary sex has been for you ever since. Maybe you feel lonely. Whatever comes up between the two of you while you make love is a way for you to connect. You need to agree that the purpose of making love is to be close, to stay connected, to be intimate with the truth of the moment. This is very different from what we are taught sex is supposed to be.

If you've seen sex as pure pleasure, as a way to escape or lose yourself for a while, it will be difficult to see that it is simply life: whatever emerges is what you work with. Sex is good when it is connected to real feelings, when you communicate, when you respond to whatever is going on, whether it's a peak of sexual arousal, a struggle to stay present, a new incest memory, or a moment when the boundaries between you dissolve.

I remember someone saying to me when I was doing intense incest work, "Everything is grist for therapy." The same is true for sex. Everything that is deep, elemental, and alive in us comes up when we make love. It is one of the ways we get in touch with our deepest selves. It's not surprising that so much emerges when we touch and touch deeply.

If sex is the only way the survivor is getting touched, it makes sense that sex is the primary way flashbacks emerge. When I was struggling with flashbacks intruding on my lovemaking, I gradually realized that sex was my only means for getting deeply in touch with my body. Through trial and error, I learned that if I found other ways to feel safe and connect deeply with myself (therapy, writing, massages, bodywork), I didn't have to store up all the memories that needed to pour out for the times I made love.

I still had flashbacks when I was making love, but not as many. Most importantly, my attitude about the flashbacks changed. Instead of telling myself, "I hate it! I'm a sexual failure. No one will ever want to be with me," I thought instead, "This hurts, Laura, but it's an opportunity to find out about your history. This is something you asked for: knowledge, validation, a better sense of what your life was like as a child." I gave myself permission to explore each flashback, to go into it and learn what it had to tell me, instead of freezing, pushing my partner away, and feeling ashamed and hopeless. When

I realized that my commitment was to staying present, and not to having "hot" sex, I didn't need to shut my partner out as much. I felt less ashamed, clearer about what I needed, and the world opened up.

Everyone in our culture has strange ideas about sex. Sex is exploited, sells products, determines our self-worth and desirability, and is used as a weapon to dominate, manipulate, humiliate, demean, and punish. This is not what sex is supposed to be. We're afraid of the real power of sex: one of the few permissible ways we have to get in touch with our most elemental selves. When we see it that way, a flashback can be just part of the experience. Lean into it, get inside it with the survivor, be a witness, stay close.

Now this is much easier to say than it is to do. Sometimes the survivor shuts you out and you can't find a way in. Or maybe you've been patient for months and you want this moment to be about you for a change. Maybe it's mindless sex you want—the good old-fashioned unconscious kind—the kind that's about your orgasm and forgetting what your boss said to you that afternoon. You don't want to pay attention to every subtle feeling the survivor has. You don't want to be sensitive. You don't want to enter into the experience with him. You want what you want and you're frustrated about not getting it. That's fine. It's the truth of your experience. You have the right to be angry, but it won't make the flashback go away. It won't make you closer or give you what you want; it'll probably create distance (at least temporarily) between the two of you. That's fine too. Your needs aren't always going to be compatible. But if you want to stay connected to the survivor, you need to be willing to enter into what is there. It may be boring, it may be horrifying, it may disgust you or move you to tears. It may not be what you want, but it's what's there.

When I'm in a workshop and a partner says he can't stand being rejected one more time, or that she just wants to have sex and stop being so damned sensitive, I look up and ask, "Do you really want to make love to someone who isn't there? Do you want to have sex with someone who is in a panic, seeing visions of being raped, or isn't there at all? Do you want to have sex with someone who is checked out, totally disconnected, hating himself, and just going through the motions?"

"I guess not," they always say.

FLASHBACKS

Sit down with a piece of paper and write down what sex is for you. Separately from you, have the survivor do the same. Include everything. Write for ten minutes and don't censor yourself. Just keep writing the sentence, "Sex is . . ." and complete each one. Some of what you write may be crazy or surprising. It doesn't matter; write whatever comes up.

Here's what one group of partners came up with:

- Sex is intimacy, love, sharing; but sometimes also control.
- Sex is misunderstood.
- Sex is wonderful and enjoyable.
- Sex is sometimes dirty, a hassle.
- I don't know what sex is.
- Sex is the highest physical expression of love.
- Sex is fun, scary, and unfulfilling.
- Sex is passionate and exciting.
- Sex is an expression of bonding, attachment, trust, and intimacy.
- Sex is highly overrated.
- Sex is a physical expression of vulnerability.
- Sex is a place where I lose control over my well-being.
- Sex is a delicate and confusing arena for shared spiritual growth.
- Sex is fun, frightening, powerful. For being a relatively small part of life, it carries a huge amount of importance.
- Sex is an area where many people have extreme expectations.
- Sex is something I have a love/hate relationship with.
- Sex is difficult to initiate.
- Sex is a wonderful or frightening experience depending on the motives of the partners. It can nurture or destroy.
- Sex is going through the motions without having any feelings.
- Sex is abuse, addiction, control, guilt, and remorse.
- Sex is a weapon; a way of destroying another human being.
- Sex is an individual experience based on knowledge gained in childhood.
- Sex is surrendering control.
- Sex is letting go; it breaks down barriers.
- Sex is overwhelming, mysterious.
- Sex is an erotic activity which includes the imagination.

- Sex is an intimate sharing of energy.
- Sex is a wonderful, scary way to share your deepest place with someone you love.
- Sex is nice, loving, comforting, good, and gone.
- Sex is an incredibly intense, positive experience to be shared by two people of equal ability to give consent.
- Sex is sometimes full of color; sometimes cold, distant, and intrusive.
- Sex is intercourse designed for the union of man and wife in marriage.
- Sex is like eating soft chocolate.
- Sex balances and releases stress.
- Sex is power, security, and identity.
- Sex is complicated, exciting, comforting, silly, hot.
- Sex is the loving physical, spiritual union of two consenting people.
- Sex is caring and sharing without thinking only of myself.
- Sex is juicy, fun, frightening, awful, and more.
- Sex is life, closeness, vulnerability, risk.
- Sex is an area of great conflict.
- Sex is the way my body expresses the love in my heart.
- Sex is only one way I connect with my partner.

Sit down with the survivor and share your lists together; it's a good way to initiate a conversation about sex. One man did this exercise with his lover. Afterward he said, "Sexuality is one of those topics I grew up not talking about. It's one of those things you grow up and learn and assume is the same for everybody. I'm finding out it isn't." Another partner concluded. "I'm probably as confused about how this sex thing works as anybody."

As you compare lists, see if you can find some small area of compatibility. The goal should be to redefine sex in your relationship; to come up with a common goal for sexual intimacy. This is a radical thing to do. Instead of coming to sex as separate people with completely different needs and expectations (usually unspoken), you'll have a common cause: "We will be awake with whatever happens when we make love (or try to). Whatever comes up, we will follow it together, and keep talking." If you can make this kind of agreement (yours can be different), you stop being adversaries. You have a shared goal that doesn't have to do with particular sexual acts or outcomes, but rather with the quality of your connection. You enter sex together as allies rather than opponents.

Being sexual with a survivor can be very hard. You may decide you don't want to grow in this particular way. You want sex to be easy: a way to connect, to simply and easily express love, to sleep better at night. That's fine. The choice is yours to make. Although it will be painful, you can leave the relationship you're in and get involved with someone who isn't trying to heal from sexual abuse. (This may be harder to find than you think.) But don't expect sex to be simple or easy with a survivor in the midst of healing. That's not possible. Healing from sexual abuse is about being awake—to both pleasure and pain. You have to decide if you're willing to go on the journey.

How do I know if a sexual experience is bringing up associations to the abuse for her? If it is, and we have to stop, what can I do about my own sexual needs?

Ask. Then ask again. Make it part of your lovemaking to kiss or touch for a while and then to ask, "Hi. How are you?" Then kiss a little longer. Explore her body. Then ask, "Are you okay? Are you still with me?"

Tune in to the survivor's body signals. Sometimes it's hard for survivors to use words to express what's going on. If you pay attention, you can usually sense a change in her body or mood when old feelings come up. Does she tense up? Stop looking at you? Close her eyes? Get stiff? Stop talking? Get still? Pout? Start acting like a child? Is there a particular moment when you start feeling like you're all alone?

When you're not in the middle of making love, talk about the things that trigger her. Devise a signal she can give you when she's in trouble: she can tap your arm in a specific, predetermined way or use a code word, like "ghosts." Discuss what she wants you to do when she signals you. Does she want you to hold her? To talk? To leave her alone for a while? See if you can find a way to stay together as she goes through the old feelings. That way, you'll feel less abandoned and disappointed, and she'll learn that she doesn't have to go through it alone. Even though you've stopped making love, try to find a way to stay connected.

Sometimes it's hard for survivors to be honest because they're afraid of disappointing you or are frightened of your anger. The survivor may hide her experience from you (and sometimes, from herself) because she believes it's her job to satisfy you sexually. (It isn't.) For her to feel safe answering your questions honestly, she has to know that it's really okay with you if she has to stop. So ask yourself, "Is it or isn't it?" If it isn't, you have some stretching to do. Unless she wants to continue, you have to learn to stop. Otherwise you'll be having sex with someone who's not there and really doesn't want to be. That's an awful lot like rape. You need to learn to stop no matter how turned on you are. No one ever died from not having an orgasm.

Ideally, you want the transition from making love to not making love to be as smooth as possible. Be as gracious as you can. (This goes for both of you.) If you throw your pillow down in disgust, jump out of bed, and storm out of the room, you only create more separation. If she turns on you and tells you you're an animal because you have sexual desires, she alienates you further. If you get caught in the trap of blaming each other, you'll only end up feeling more isolated and alone.

Find a way to stay close when you have to stop in the middle of making love. Don't turn away into your private pain. Remind yourself: "This isn't easy for either of us. We're both hurting." If you find a way to bridge to another way of connecting (holding her while she cries, she holding you while you touch yourself, getting out of bed and going for a walk), having to stop won't seem like such an abrupt failure.

Sometimes this isn't possible. The survivor is withdrawn and doesn't know how to reach out. You're furious (this is the fifteenth time in a row) and you care about your release, not her damn memories! If you're that far apart, don't try to bridge to another activity. Spend some time apart, take care of your conflicting needs, and then come back together and talk about what happened.

As far as your own unfulfilled sexual needs, you're going to have to masturbate a lot more than usual. (I know, I know. It's not the same. It's the survivor you really want.) With the right attitude, self-stimulation can be erotic and fun. Other times, when you're feeling rejected, masturbation will feel lonely and sad. Touching yourself can bring up feelings of sorrow that you can't have sex the way you want to.

Sometimes survivors are willing to participate while you touch yourself. Maybe the survivor can't stimulate you sexually (or let you touch her), but perhaps she can hold you (or watch) while you masturbate. Although some survivors can't handle any kind of sexual arousal, even at a distance, others can. Ask. Experiment. The survivor might surprise you with her willingness and creativity, as long as she knows you'll respect her limits.

Is it okay to share my feelings of disappointment and rejection when my lover can't be sexual? He already knows how I feel and feels badly. It feels like rubbing his nose in something he can't do differently. But in the moment, I hurt and swallow it down.

It's absolutely natural for you to feel let down and frustrated when you have to stop in the middle of making love. But if you express your anger, sadness, and frustration just when the survivor is deep into a memory, you'll become even more alienated from each other.

Wait until you're out of the situation to express how difficult it was for you. And don't do all the expressing with the survivor. He may not be able to handle the full weight of your feelings: he feels guilty enough already for having said no in the first place. He's struggling with his own sense of failure and isn't the right person to hear the full depth of your frustration.

On the other hand, the survivor needs to know how you feel. He needs to tell you, with sincerity and caring, that he's sorry you're having such a hard time. And most important, you need to hear him say, repeatedly, that he's committed to working this through so that things can change. His words won't take your pain away, or put your immediate needs in alignment, but they can make a tremendous difference in the way you feel.

Whatever you do, don't swallow your feelings. You have a right to feel exasperated, sad, abandoned, lonely, and angry. Express those feelings fully. Pound a few pillows. Go to the gym and work up a sweat. Cry on your way to work. Talk to other people who care about you. Remind yourself that this is the abuser's fault. Write the @#%$# a hate letter. (You don't have to send it.) Buy yourself a medal of valor. Then come back to the survivor in the spirit of willingness, to work with what's actually there.

How can I integrate my sexuality with the survivor's when there are such profound and dramatic differences in our sexual needs?

Finding common sexual ground with a survivor takes communication, honesty, and compromise. (And if you're with a survivor anywhere near the beginning of the healing process, it's likely that a vast majority of the compromise in this area will be yours.) The places your sexual interests intersect may be very small right now—you want to have orgasmic sex and the survivor can't bear to be touched. But even when your capabilities and needs seem opposed, you can still be united in a desire to build, over time, a shared sexual life together.

A good way to explore your sexual common ground is through the use of safe sex guidelines. I first introduced these in *The Courage to Heal Workbook*.[1] Survivors fill out a chart which divides sexual/sensual activities into three categories: Safe, Possibly Safe, and Unsafe. Safe sex activities are those body-related pleasures that are comfortable and free from associations to abuse. Unsafe activities are things that inevitably bring up fear, bad feelings, and memories of abuse. Possibly Safe activities are in the middle—sometimes they're okay; sometimes they trigger difficult feelings from the past. In making these lists, I ask survivors to use as broad a definition of sex as possible—to include things they can do alone or with a partner; things traditionally considered "sexual" and things that are more sensual in nature. Anything connected with pleasurable feelings in their bodies is included. The idea is for survivors to start their sexual exploration by limiting themselves to the activities that are safe for them. That way, instead of continually facing failure, they can build up a store of positive experiences with sex.

What survivors consider safe and unsafe varies widely—one survivor loves bathing with candles, and puts it at the top of his safe list. Another, who was abused in the bathtub, puts it firmly in the unsafe category. Some survivors have many activities listed in their safe category; others struggle to find just one or two. For many, the safe

---

[1] Laura Davis, *The Courage to Heal Workbook*, p. 440.

activities are more sensual than sexual in nature—holding hands, dancing, flirting, petting kittens, eating by candlelight, curling up in bed with a fluffy down comforter. But this isn't always true. Some survivors find gentle, tender touch and cuddling much more threatening than stimulating a partner to orgasm. There are no right answers in filling out safe sex guidelines. They are there to help survivors identify negative triggers and to give them a safe place to begin.

Filling out safe sex guidelines along with the survivor is an excellent way to explore common ground. Although you may not think about sexual or sensual activities as safe or unsafe, you can probably categorize activities by levels of comfort: Most Comfortable, Usually Comfortable, Least Comfortable. Or try: Most Preferred, Generally Fine, Least Preferred. If these categories don't feel right to you, make up your own classifications. Put your headings at the top of a blank sheet of paper, draw a column under each one, and take fifteen minutes to fill them in. (It's okay if things get sandwiched between two categories. Things aren't always so black and white.)

When partners do this exercise, they're often surprised (and actually relieved) to realize that there are some sexual things they like better than others. Others realize that they really do prefer sensuality to the pressure to perform sexually. Many are surprised that they've been doing things for years that they're really not all that comfortable with.

Once you've finished your list, sit down with the survivor and compare what you've each come up with. It may be that there are several things on the "safe" or "comfortable" list that you share. (Or things that are on his safe list that you can add to yours, and vice versa.) If that's the case, you've just identified the areas in which you can physically and sensually be close right now. There may not be many, but at least things are clearer between you. You may feel bad about giving up some of the activities you love (at least for now), but you weren't actually sharing them successfully anyway. When you know what's possible and what isn't, you won't keep feeling rejected asking for something the survivor is not able to give.

If there isn't any common ground between you right now, it may be that this is the time the survivor needs to take a break from sex (see page 182) or needs to explore his body and his sexuality on his own. Although this may be difficult for you, at least you know what is going on and are free to make a conscious decision to support your partner. Even if you feel deprived, you can feel deprived knowing that you are doing something genuinely helpful. You are taking an action that will make things better in the long run. That's better than being caught in a power struggle or trying to engage in sex that only makes things worse. Even if a moratorium on sex is not your first choice (or your second or your third), it may well be the first step toward a future of shared physical closeness between you.

Unfortunately, as the partner of a survivor, you are the one who has to put your sexual needs on hold. The survivor's need to feel safe and in control has to take precedence. It takes a long time for survivors to feel secure enough in their ownership of their own sexuality to allow you to assert yourself more. Although survivors eventually can get to the point where they can begin to respond to your needs and your desires, this doesn't happen until much later in the sexual healing process—sometimes years later. I know this is difficult to accept, but it's important to be realistic. Sexual healing is very slow. The survivor is not going to transform overnight; then again, neither are you. But if you begin where you are and keep working individually and together, you can make steady progress toward a mutual sexual life you can share.

Even if the survivor can't meet you halfway, not by a long shot, it would be nice, at a minimum, for him to appreciate you for what you're doing. He can say, "I know this is very hard for you. I'm sorry. I really appreciate your willingness to hang in here with me." He can grow to respect you and your sexual feelings, instead of seeing them as a threat: "There's nothing wrong with your sexuality. I admire it. And one day I hope I can meet it fully." He can tell you that he shares your vision of one day having a sexual life that is freely chosen and freely shared. He can take active steps to keep moving forward in his own healing. And of course, he can write you love notes.

I hear partners complain all the time about not getting enough sex. I have the opposite problem. My lover wants to have sex all the time. It feels like the sex has very little to do with being close to me. I end up feeling used. She's had affairs, too. I've been hurt by her repeatedly. What's going on?

Many survivors withdraw from sex and are frightened by it. Others learn to use sex as their primary way of moving through the world. As a child, performing sexually may have been the one way the survivor was loved, appreciated, and valued. Now, she equates sex with love. Being "good at sex" is a way for her to feel good about herself.

She may have also learned that sex was a way to control people. Being able to elicit a sexual response gave her a sense of power. Sex became a tool of manipulation. If she wanted to control someone, she learned to incite their desire. She learned to play the role of "temptress," luring people in sexually, and then casting them away. In this scenario, anyone who responded to her was seen as weak, or even pitiful.

This pattern of involvement doesn't necessarily end because the survivor got involved with you. She may still have trouble bridging sexuality and intimacy. Sex may still be her primary coping strategy; her main way to meet her needs. She may not respect you if you desire her sexually; she may be using sex to manipulate, punish, or control you.

For this pattern to change, the survivor needs to learn that sex, caring, and vulnerability can go together. She needs to find other ways to meet her basic needs—asking for appreciation or holding, for instance, instead of sex. She also needs to look at the ways she's been hurt by sex and to acknowledge the ways she's used sex to hurt others. When her sexual bravado is peeled back, a frightened little girl may emerge.

Survivors who are highly sexual are not exempt from the need for sexual healing. When a survivor has used sex as a primary identity and honestly begins to explore the underlying reasons, her sexuality can be radically affected. She may not be able to be sexual in the ways she was before. She may need to shut down and say no to sex for a time.

If the survivor has hurt you through her sexual behavior, you're going to have to assess the weight of that hurt. Has your trust been shattered irrevocably? Do you feel so violated you need to walk away? Is there anything the survivor could do to regain your trust? What do you need to do to heal the hurts you've suffered?

The fact that the survivor was abused as a child doesn't give her license to hurt you. Understanding her history may help you understand her actions, but it doesn't mean you have to condone them or allow them to continue. If you stay in the relationship, talk about the ways you've been hurt. Set limits about the kinds of behavior you will and won't accept. Establish ground rules. Talk about the kind of relationship you want to have. If the survivor is willing to take responsibility for the ways she's hurt you, you'll have a chance of working things out. If she doesn't, there'll be little chance of reestablishing the trust and safety necessary to establish a sexual relationship on more solid, mutual ground.

How can I convince my wife that sex isn't my biggest concern?

Survivors sometimes assume that men only want sex because of what they were taught about boys and men. One partner explained:

> What my wife was told by her father, and what her father demonstrated to her, was that men were sexually out of control. Boys had one thing in mind and that was a sexual objective. He told her that boys were ruled by their penises and could in no way control what they did. The girl's job was to say no. Boys weren't allowed upstairs in her house, because basically, the sight of a bed would drive them completely out of control. They had to stay in the kitchen when they visited. And of course, he backed this up with his own behavior. He couldn't keep his hands off her. So when we got involved, she assumed I also was just another sexually out of control man. Even if I said to her, "We can just lie here and cuddle. I don't have to have an orgasm," she never really believed me. She never trusted me not to be secretly concerned with my "final objective."

When a woman has been conditioned to think about men this way, she needs to have a different experience to counter her preconceptions. When you appreciate her, make sure you appreciate her for things other than her looks and her sex appeal. Be warm and loving and affectionate at times when you're not approaching her for sex.

Let her know that you can be sexually aroused and not satisfied by her, and that you won't die from it. You may feel frustrated or disappointed, but you'll live. Remind her you respect her right and need to say no. Say no yourself sometimes. (But not as a way to get even with her.)

Also, take a look at your own responses and attitudes. How do you respond when she turns you down? Do you sulk, withdraw, or otherwise punish her when she says no? These kinds of behaviors can subtly reinforce her belief that you're really trying to manipulate her into sex.

Practice other ways the two of you can be intimate. Make dates to do things that make you feel close. Agree to keep sex out of it and stick with the boundaries you set. If you let these activities lead to sex, you'll reinforce the message that sex is really your ultimate goal. If you consistently do things that create intimacy without sex as the outcome, she'll gradually see that you're "not the same as all the other men." (For more on the problem of gender stereotyping, see page 130.)

Ultimately your integrity is going to have to speak for itself. (See "Trust" on page 153.) If you consistently demonstrate that you're not just interested in sex, and she still isn't seeing you for who you are, but as "Generic Man," tell her you don't like it and that your feelings are hurt. No one wants to be treated like a sexual monster. Let her know you feel stereotyped and invisible. Knowing that she's hurting you may help her take a more realistic look at who you really are.

Why does the survivor find violent sexual fantasies so provocative?

When children are sexually abused a certain imprinting takes place. The child is bombarded with a variety of sensations—sexual arousal, terror, love, physical pain, humiliation, shame, and confusion. These sensations and feelings get imprinted together. They get intertwined. A young boy is beaten with a belt every night by his father, who then climbs into bed with the boy and stimulates him sexually. The child learns to associate violence, the fear of violence, the sensation of being hit, and the cessation of the hitting, with sexual arousal. This linkage is created for him and as an adult, he associates the two—sex and violence. He masturbates to violent pornography or feels turned on after a fight.

Adult survivors frequently need to recreate the feelings they had as children, when they first were sexually stimulated, in order to be sexually aroused. As a result, many adult survivors have violent or sadistic fantasies, get involved in sadomasochism, or put themselves in situations where sex is linked with danger, secrecy, humiliation, or violence. Many secretly masturbate when they read or hear about incest. This recreates aspects of the abuse and reinforces the linkage. The survivor may have experiences like these and keep them a shameful secret. He may not be able to admit to you, or even to himself, what he really experiences sexually. It's less painful to just shut down. However, to heal sexually, these patterns eventually have to be acknowledged, accepted for what they are, and gradually broken down.

Other survivors experience the linkage this way: they feel aroused, and instantly the old feelings crowd in. Instead of feeling open, receptive, and loving when they are touched, they feel disgusted and dirty and want to throw up. They feel terrified, humiliated, ashamed, and confused; this mirrors their experience as children. This is one of the primary reasons survivors shut down sexually and feel ashamed of their sexual feelings.

Many times, too, survivors believe their bodies betrayed them when they were children: they responded sexually to abuse. This is one of the deepest pockets of shame many survivors carry. As a boy, the survivor tried to stop himself from getting an erection or having an orgasm, but his body responded; he believes his experience of pleasure made the abuse his fault. This is not true. Our bodies are designed to respond to stimulation. If an abuser wants a child to have an orgasm, get an erection, or become aroused, he or she can stimulate the child to make it happen. It's one of the ways abusers exert power and control over their victims: stimulating a child to orgasm is an effective way of reinforcing the child's sense of compliance, shame, and silence.

As a partner it can be difficult to understand this. If the survivor had an orgasm, you may secretly wonder if he really liked the abuse; if it really was all that bad. You don't understand why the survivor has so many painful associations to pleasure; when you are sexually aroused, you feel whole, happy, connected to yourself. Many survivors experience the opposite: arousal doesn't feel good to them. Rather than feel the scary, confusing sensations and memories that accompany sex for them, they shut down. Think about it from the survivor's point of view: Would you want to make love if sex made you feel ashamed, disgusted, and self-hating?

It is possible to undo this kind of early conditioning, to disconnect the linkage between violence, humiliation, pain, and sex. But the survivor needs to be ready to do it. Changing body associations is slow, painstaking work. For excellent, practical suggestions on changing negative associations to sex, read *The Sexual Healing Journey* by Wendy Maltz. (See the bibliography for details.)

My wife says she thinks she might be a lesbian. I don't know what to do with this information.

The news that your partner is questioning his or her sexual orientation is hard to hear, to say the least. You probably feel confused, bewildered, and threatened. (Unless you're in denial about the whole thing, in which case you're probably not feeling anything.) When your partner says he or she may really be homosexual (or heterosexual, depending on your orientation), you're bound to feel powerless. After all, you're pretty much stuck with the gender you've got. If the survivor decides to stop having relationships with men (or women, as the case might be), the survivor is going to stop having a relationship with you. That's about as personal as you can get.

Before I talk about what you face as a partner in this situation, I'd like to explain my perspective on sexual orientation. To begin with, I'm a lesbian. I feel good about being a lesbian. I don't think there's anything wrong with being gay or lesbian. (I don't think there's anything wrong with being heterosexual or bisexual either.) I march in the gay pride parade every year with my heterosexual father and I'm proud of who I am. I make a point of coming out whenever I make a public presentation. I want people to see me and know that all lesbians are not _____ (fill in the blank with your favorite stereotype). Because I come out in public, and tell people I'm willing to talk about it, I always get asked, "Are you a lesbian because you were abused?"

I always answer the same way: "No." Depending on my audience, I sometimes add my favorite quote from a very articulate incest survivor: "If I'm a lesbian because I was sexually abused, at least something good came out of it." Or I say to the audience, "Think about the number of women in this country who have been sexually abused by men. If sexual abuse was the determining factor in creating lesbians, the lesbian population would be far greater than it is today."[1]

Sexual orientation is best seen on a continuum. Some people are exclusively heterosexual; some exclusively homosexual. Most are

---

[1] From *The Courage to Heal*, p. 268.

somewhere in-between. If our society wasn't so terrified of homosexuality and didn't come down so hard on people for same-sex attractions, there'd be a lot more variation in the way most of us live.

No one has yet come up with a definitive reason why some people are heterosexual and some homosexual. There is no proof that more women become lesbians or men become gay because they were sexually abused as children. (There are plenty of gay men and lesbians who *weren't* abused as children, too.) I have noticed, however, that a higher proportion of lesbians and gay men have stepped forward to say that they were abused. I think this is indicative of: (a) the fact that lesbians have less reason to protect men, and a majority of abusers are men; (b) there's more support in the gay and lesbian community for exploring these issues; and (c) gay men and lesbians have actively looked at their sexuality in order to come out in the first place; because of this increased awareness, there's more of an opportunity for them to stumble upon the information that they were sexually abused.

One thing I have observed through my years of work with survivors is that many of them, whether gay, straight, or bisexual, go through a period where they question, and sometimes shift, their sexual orientation. In some instances, this questioning arises from misinformation: "Boys become homosexual when they are sexually abused by men. I am gay and I must be gay because my uncle had sex with me." Other times, it comes from internalized homophobia[2]: "I'm a lesbian. There must be something wrong with me because I'm a lesbian. To be healthy, I have to change." The question may also arise from a generalization: "I was abused by a man. No men are trustworthy. Therefore, I need to be with women." Or from a false belief: "My relationships with men are so hard. If I become a lesbian, things will magically change and my relationships will be wonderful." Many survivors wonder about their sexual orientation because they never got to ask the question before. They were too busy being sexually abused to explore their own sexual feelings. At thirteen, when other little boys were growing interested in girls (or secretly, in other little boys), the survivor was too busy fending off his brothers to know who he was drawn to. He never had a chance to ask the question, and now he wants to know.

---

[2] Homophobia is the fear and hatred of homosexuality and homosexuals.

In the course of healing, many survivors need to go through those early, missed stages of sexual development all over again. They need the freedom to ask: "Who do I want to be with? What is my real nature?" I encourage survivors to ask themselves these questions and to explore. I say, "Spend time with people who will not try to influence you either way. Take your time. Eventually, you will know what's right for you."

Of course, if the survivor is already in a committed, intimate relationship with you, this questioning process will be very hard to take. Let's look at it from your point of view: You've already invested years in your relationship. You have children, a home, a life together. You've been patient and supportive through months (or years) of this incest crap, and now she thinks she's a lesbian? For you, this is the last straw. You want to scream at her, "How can you do this to me?"

This brings us back to our original question: What do you do, as a partner, when your lover says he or she may be shifting orientations?

Unfortunately, there are no easy answers. During this exploratory stage, the survivor may, in fact, be uncovering his or her real sexual orientation. Or things could go the other way: if you hold steady and step back, the survivor's explorations may lead to the conclusion that he or she is already in the right place. There's no predicting what's going to happen.

What's imperative is that you get support. You need someone to talk to. You may feel like you've been duped or used; you may feel a deep sense of betrayal or inadequacy. You need to talk about your fears, insecurities, and anger. It's unfortunate that you're in this situation, but unless you're ready to walk out today, you need to learn to live with the ambiguity for a while. Reach out. Don't try to sit with this alone.

If you and the survivor ultimately do split over this, it doesn't mean you're not lovable or desirable. It means that you were in a relationship where differing needs moved you in opposite directions. That's a personal tragedy for you, but it doesn't mean you're jinxed, or that someone else won't love you.

How do I reconcile my need for a good sexual relationship with the survivor's fear of sex? At what point do I give up hope of resolving this, if I am not willing to be in a long-term asexual relationship?

The answers to the questions in this section have given you an accurate picture of what you're up against in a sexual relationship with a survivor. Although all survivors are different (and are at different stages in their healing), certain commonalities do exist. If you and the survivor are having troubles with sex, or are not having sex at all, there are certain steps you will both have to go through for things to change.

It is definitely possible to experience sexual healing in a relationship with a survivor. But it can only happen if and when the survivor is ready. He has to want to work on sexual issues for his own reasons. If he doesn't, positive change can't occur. Even if he's willing and ready, change will be very slow.

So, if you're wondering whether you should stick it out, there are some questions you need to address honestly: "Is sexual healing something the survivor is ready and willing to tackle at this time?" "How patient can I be?" "Am I committed enough to this relationship to accept delayed gratification of one of my most basic needs?" "What price will I pay if I stay?" "What are the potential benefits if I see it through?" "Am I willing to take the risk that it won't work out or that the survivor will leave me in the end?"

There is nothing wrong with you for wanting to have a relationship that includes sex. You are not a lower form of life because you don't want a celibate partnership. You're entitled to want and have sexual sharing. What you have to take into account is the rest of your life —your family, your children, the other aspects of your relationship that are rewarding and worthwhile. Ask yourself: "What would things be like between us if sex wasn't an issue? Would they still be rocky?" "How would my life change if I left?" "How would I feel?" "When I look at the whole picture, where does sex (or lack of sex) fit in?"

Bill, a partner with young children at home, described his struggles over this issue with his wife, Sharon:

Sharon needs a lot of things to feel secure in a sexual surrounding: things that are calming and soothing; the feeling that there are no expectations or demands. At first I said, "Yes, I can do this. I'm altruistic enough." I was very giving and self-sacrificing. But then the door would slam shut again. It made me feel terrible.

I'm a person who deals with life on a sensual level. I'm into food and cooking; I'm into touch. This was not an area of my adult life where I expected to be shortchanged or denied. Feeling robbed makes it hard for me to say, "This is great. This is you and I love this about you." That's the thing she wants me to say: "I love everything about you, including the fact that you were abused as a child and the difficulties it presents for you as an adult." I haven't been able to say that. I say, "I hate this. I can't stand the fact that I can't come to bed at night, give you a hug, and be met with a warm feeling. Every time I touch you, your initial response is fear." At her best, Sharon says, "I'm doing well because I'm sort of enjoying myself. I'm not having flashbacks; I don't feel like I have a knife in my solar plexus." That wears away at me.

I've been very angry, but it's been hard for me to tell her how frustrated I am without feeling I'm hurting or attacking her. When I tell her, "I feel so deprived of the opportunity to express my sexuality, to develop myself as a sexual being," her response is usually, "I'm a horrible person. You should leave me or I should kill myself." She has felt at times that I should leave because I'd never be happy with her, and at times, I've agreed.

I've thought about giving up on the relationship. I don't really permit myself to think about that now. I can't imagine splitting up while we have kids. The main problem in the relationship is sex and that's not enough of a reason to end the relationship. We have so many other wonderful things between us. I love my family. I love having kids. Sharon's a great mother. Yet I'd love it for the whole thing to go away. When I get into bed, my thoughts are often, "I can't believe this is the situation I'm in." I've accepted it, although not happily.

Leaving a relationship because you are not sexually satisfied is a big step. It's not one to take hastily. If you're thinking about leaving, make sure you've had a chance to talk to survivors and partners who've made it through the hard times to a place where they feel good about sex again. You need role models to know it's possible, and safe places to talk things through. Skilled people can guide you through the sexual healing process and give you a sense of what to expect. Beyond that, only you know your own breaking point. (See page 87 for more on deciding whether to leave or stay).

FAMILY ISSUES

"I'd walk around and see pictures of her at her mom's house. In every picture, I'd see a terrified little girl. She's never smiling in those pictures. She has this look that just says, 'Someone, please come help me.' It makes me feel really angry at her parents."

"Being a father has been an incredibly healing force for him. He loves the kids and feels proud that we've broken the cycle of abuse."

My wife has all kinds of mixed feelings about her father. I don't understand how she could still love him. He raped her! I hate him and she feels threatened by that. What should I do?

When someone you love has been sexually abused by someone in her family, you have the right to be furious. As one partner put it, "There are times I've gotten really angry at her father. Not just because he abused and tortured her, but because he screwed up our lives, probably for the rest of our lives."

You don't have to like the abuser. You don't have to feel anything but your authentic feelings about him. If you think he's a miserable rotten slime, that's okay. As one partner explained, he probably is: "I never liked her father. He was an intolerable, nasty human being. He clearly was unhappy with his life. He wasn't deriving any joy from being alive."

If, however, the survivor is not yet in touch with her anger (or it's too mixed in with love and confusion), it's important that you don't overwhelm her with your strong, unbridled emotions. This is a place where the line between your feelings and hers is very important. While you can model what healthy (and appropriate) anger at the abuser looks like, it's important that she have the room to explore her own feelings at her own pace. Things may not be as clear for her as they are for you. This man who abused her is the only father she'll ever have; it's painful for her to acknowledge that he hurt her and didn't have her best interests at heart. For her, such an admission represents a very primal loss: her daddy didn't take care of his little girl. Whether the survivor is twenty or sixty, this knowledge is excruciating.

Survivors rarely feel one way toward their perpetrators, particularly when the abuser is a family member. Most feel some combination of love, anguish, hatred, rage, confusion, fear, loyalty, and longing. This is natural. Even when they are treated terribly, children hold on to the hope that they can change things by altering their own behavior. This unrealistic wish demonstrates the extent to which children will twist things so they don't have to see the adults around them as unreliable, hurtful, or out of control.

Adult children often continue to protect abusers by rationalizing the abusers' behavior or blaming themselves. "He'd just come back from the war. It must have been the stress of the war," one survivor told me. Her father had violently raped her and left her for dead when she was three years old. Another man tried to convince me the abuse was his fault. "I was a needy kid," he told me, with all sincerity. "I wanted my father to hold me. If I hadn't gone in for that hug, it never would have happened."

Survivors would rather do anything than place the responsibility where it belongs. It's too painful to face the loss.

The survivor may also be struggling with mixed feelings toward the abuser because her memories of abuse are mixed with happier memories. Many abusers also show love and caring to their victims. The same man who raped the survivor may have patiently taught her to ride a bike or brought her special books from the library. He may have been the only person who ever treated her like she was special. Although this doesn't excuse him, it does help explain why the survivor's feelings are so conflicted now. It may take years for her to sort through her mixed emotions. She needs that time. She needs room to test things out with the abuser (and other family members), to try yet again to change things, to find her way through trial and error. It's only by repeatedly going through the cycle of loss, anger, disappointment, and revised expectations that a survivor reaches a place of resolution in her feelings toward her family. Even then, circumstances shift and things change.

All this time you may be very clear about your feelings. You know how you feel about the abuser: You hate the guy. You want revenge. You can't stand watching the survivor get hurt by her family over and over again. It's painful to see her get her hopes smashed repeatedly. You ache to protect her from this kind of disappointment. You want to do something to make it better, to clear things up once and for all.

You can't.

Although you can support her, listen to her, and provide a sounding board, the survivor has to sort out her own relationship with her abuser and her family. Expect her feelings to change over time. That doesn't mean yours have to. (For more on emotional boundaries, see pages 72 and 81.)

When do you get over losing your in-laws?

You may never get over the loss entirely. A thread, a sense of trust has been broken. If you had a close relationship with your in-laws, and then found out they abused, failed to protect, or deeply hurt your partner, it can be hard to reconcile that information with your love for them. If the survivor needs you to curtail your relationship with them, it will be a difficult loss, one you will have to grieve. But abuse has its consequences, both in your life and in theirs: the schism in your relationship is the natural consequence of abuse.

Try not to get upset with the survivor. Respect her need to separate and support whatever decisions she needs to make. Her needs regarding her parents take precedence over yours. If you still have positive, loving feelings toward your in-laws and want to continue a social relationship with them, and the survivor doesn't want you to, you'll have to put your feelings aside in order to respect her wishes. Dealing with the survivor's family is one of the ways you're more directly affected by the abuse. Her loss is your loss. As one partner put it:

> Whatever she wants in terms of contact with them, she's the one in charge. I feel really comfortable with that. I completely support her. But detaching from her family has been really sad for me. My family lives across the country. I miss my family, and I'd like to be close to her family. I like her family. But with the molestation, it's not possible. Her parents like to come to the city and go out to dinner, and we can't do that with them. They go to Hawaii and stay in a condo where there'd be an extra room for us, and we can never go. Her mom knows how to can food, and I'd love to learn how to do that, but we can't go out there. There's a lot of loss involved.

However you handle the loss, don't blame the survivor for taking your in-laws away. See if you can grieve together instead.

I have a strong desire to confront my husband's step-father myself. I feel that he needs to "pay" for what he did. What should I do?

As a partner, it's natural to desire confrontation and revenge. However, it's essential that you stand back and let the survivor initiate any confrontation with the abuser. If you confront for the survivor, you do him a great disservice. You give him the message that you don't trust him to take care of himself. You disrespect his feelings, his needs, and his sense of timing. You force him to deal with the repercussions of disclosure in his family before he's ready. Although you may feel relieved to unburden yourself, you disempower the survivor.

Certainly you need to express your anger. Go ahead. Express it. Write confrontational letters to the abuser. (But don't send them.) Indulge in revenge fantasies as much as you want. Think about how the abuser would look and sound dipped in boiling oil. Devise new and creative ways to humiliate him in public. Make each new fantasy as graphic and satisfying as possible. (This can be an enjoyable evening's activity for your partners' group.) Fantasize to your heart's content, but don't act out your fantasies. If you're bound and determined to take action, take action against abusers in general. Make a donation to an organization that's fighting child abuse, become an activist, fight to strengthen the laws against pedophiles.

Sometimes survivors do want their partners to speak up on their behalf. If you're willing to do this, offer your services: "If you ever want me to, I'd be more than happy to . . . (call him up/write her a letter/go over there and do it with you)." But make it an open-ended offer, not a declaration that you're on your way to the abuser's house. That way the survivor will feel supported rather than pressured into taking a stand he's not yet ready to take.

What's the purpose of a confrontation? Is there any way I can help?

Confronting the abuser can be a dramatic and effective way for survivors to express their anger, let go, and move on. At some point, all survivors need to confront the abuser, either symbolically (in a letter, in a role-playing situation, etc.) or directly. In a direct confrontation, survivors stand up as adults and face the person who hurt them the most. They say, "This is what you did to me. This is how it's affected me. This is how I feel about it. Here's what I want (or don't want) from you." Armed with the power and strength of the truth, survivors confront from a powerful position.

Confronting can be liberating, but also very painful. Survivors have to give up unrealistic fantasies of reconciliation. ("He'll get down on his knees, tell me he's sorry, and offer to pay for my therapy") and accept painful realities ("My father didn't apologize; my mother doesn't believe me; my brother thinks it's no big deal"). Such losses are agonizing. As one survivor put it so well, "I felt rotten before I did it, I felt rotten while I was doing it, and I felt rotten after I did it, but at least it's not hanging over my head anymore."

Some survivors choose not to confront directly. They're sick of being denied, called liars, or ignored. Their abusers may be violent, unpredictable, dead, or otherwise unavailable. It's fine to confront indirectly. Symbolic confrontations can be equally powerful.

If the survivor is considering a confrontation, it's important that she take time to prepare, plan, and think through what she's going to do and say. She needs to bring her expectations more in line with the responses she's likely to face. As a partner, you can provide some of the essential back-up support she'll need before, during, and after the confrontation.

In any confrontation, the survivor is the producer and director: she writes the script and sets the action. You work behind the scenes to make her plan possible; you're the supporting cast. Let her have center stage. This is her abuse and her abuser. Ask her if she wants help. Ask what she wants you to do. Does she want you to rehearse with her at home? To listen in on the extension when she makes the call? To go along as an ally and witness? To pick up the pieces when it's over? To be part of a symbolic confrontation?

Assisting in a confrontation is one place you can offer the survivor concrete, practical help. Your back-up support and caring can make a tremendous difference. As much as you can, give her the support she asks for.*

---

* For concrete help in planning a confrontation, see *The Courage to Heal Workbook*, pages 340–366.

What can we do when the abuser denies or justifies her actions?

Abusers universally deny abuse. They say things like "You're crazy. That never happened," or justify their actions by saying, "I was just educating my girls." It is rare for abusers to come forward with genuine grief and sorrow for their actions; they rarely face the fact that they have abused unless they are forced to go through arrest and criminal prosecution. (And even then, their denial often remains intact.)

If you're used to dealing with people who acknowledge their mistakes and work to make up for them, dealing with an abuser can be infuriating. But if you can anticipate the way most abusers react, your expectations will be more realistic: Abusers generally deny, cover up, minimize, attack, and protect themselves from the accusations any way they can.

The purpose of a confrontation is for the survivor to speak the truth; to share her hurt, outrage, and pain; to stand up as an adult and face the person who hurt her as a child. The success of a confrontation should be gauged by the survivor's courage, determination, and follow-through, not by a particular outcome or response from the abuser. Part of preparing for a confrontation is giving up the fantasy that the abuser will have a sudden, miraculous personality change. She probably won't.

In the rare circumstances where an abuser takes responsibility for her actions and genuinely tries to make amends, the survivor has to decide how to handle her gestures. Abusers often continue to manipulate survivors even when they're supposedly helping (offering to pay for therapy but then always sending the checks late). A miniscule amount of effort by the abuser is often viewed as a monumental step, worthy of the survivor's undying gratitude: "I said I was sorry if anything I did ever hurt you. What more do you want?" The survivor may want a lot more. She may want her mother to stop kissing her on the lips, making comments about her weight, or talking about sex in the living room. Actions speak a lot louder than words. Don't be taken in by a token gesture.

Even when the abuser genuinely feels bad, takes responsibility, and is respectful in her attitudes and actions today, the survivor still gets to set limits that feel good to her. She can opt not to see or talk to the abuser again, continue telling people what the abuser did, or make the choice to see if a healthier relationship is possible. The choice is always with the survivor.

BEING A MIRROR

Sometimes my wife begins defending her family and she presents an idealized picture of them. What should I do? Listen? Give feedback about what I see? Get angry? I'm not sure what helps.

The best thing for you to do is to provide an accurate mirror of what you see taking place in the survivor's family. Give her feedback about the reality you see unfolding. Don't fight about it; try to keep your responses simple, clear, and unemotional as possible. You provide a marker, a reminder of the truth. Your knowledge of the situation generally is steadier than hers; her vantage point is more likely to be clouded by emotion, longing, and denial. One partner explained:

> She's had to reconsider every single message she's gotten from her family—that they were okay, that they were decent people; everybody in the community liked them. And everything is shattering. I see walls shatter every day. It wasn't a perfect family. It was all pretend.

Having illusions about your family shattered is devastating. There will be times when the survivor needs to back off from the painful truth to give herself a break from the wrenching sense of loss. Be sensitive to this. Sometimes it's best just to listen; other times you can slip in a reality check: "Remember last month when your brother called you in the middle of the night screaming about what a liar you were? Now he's being sweet. It's just the seduction phase of the cycle; next comes the annihilation phase. We've been through this before." Or, "In the four days of her visit, your sister never once asked how you were and she cut you off every time you tried to tell her. I hardly call that a supportive relationship."

Sometimes the survivor will get mad at you for contradicting her current view of reality. "He really didn't abuse me." "My sister really has my best interests at heart." If you find yourself arguing with the survivor, back off. You've gotten trapped in a power struggle. She's defending her family; you're attacking them. You've become polarized. The painful truth you're expressing is more than she can absorb right now. Stop. Let her have her feelings.

Sometimes you can deflect an argument about her family if you clarify your motives. Tell the survivor you're saying these things because you don't like to see her turn her anger around and hate herself. It's painful for you to watch her set herself up for more disappointment. You want to protect her from being fully open to her family's violations. You care about her and want her to learn to protect herself. You provide support, strength, and clarity for the survivor by giving her honest, gentle feedback about her family. It's a tangible way to show your concern.

My lover's parents are coming to visit tomorrow. He's not ready to rock the boat by saying no to them. I respect his feelings, but I don't want to see them myself. Is it okay for me to leave?

This is a situation where there isn't a right or wrong choice. Survivors often want their partners to be around when family members visit (to act as witnesses; to give feedback, support, and encouragement), but partners sometimes have to say no based on their own needs. Many factors are involved: the partners' relationship to the parents, the history of the situation, the intensity of the partners' feelings. Some partners are comfortable putting their own feelings aside to offer support to the survivor; others aren't. One partner explained:

> She really wanted me to go with her to visit her family and I said no. I just couldn't be around her family and act like everything was normal. I could support her on the periphery—go down with her and see her afterwards, but I didn't want to be in their house with them. I hate her father too much. I just want to strangle him."

There are valid reasons for not wanting to participate in a visit with the survivor's family: pretending things are fine makes you sick to your stomach; you feel so angry you couldn't be civil if you tried; you want to kill his mother and might act on it if you were in the same room. You don't want your children in the same house as the abuser, so you plan to take them out for the day. That's a concrete way to support the survivor, whether he sees it that way or not. (See page 224 for more on protecting children.)

If you choose not to take part in the actual visit, there are still ways you can support the survivor. Help him come up with a plan for taking care of himself. Help him set goals for the visit. Check in by phone or slip out together for a couple of hours.

Survivors often forget they can set limits with abusers or family members. There's often this limp feeling of surrender. "Because I'm not ready to confront, I can't say no to anything. They can walk all over me and I can't stop them." Help the survivor fight this belief. Talk to him about ways he can start setting limits.

He may not be ready to confront his parents, for instance, but he may be able to limit the length of their visit or ask them to stay in a motel. Just because they've stayed in your house before doesn't mean they automatically have to stay there this time. Helping him think these things through beforehand can be a tremendous support, even if you choose not to be there during the actual visit.

If, on the other hand, you feel willing and able to participate in a family visit, your presence can be invaluable: you can help gather information, give objective feedback, remind the survivor to stick to his goals, and hold him at night. You can even have secret signals you use to remind him to breathe or to stick up for himself.

Either way, you can be supportive. Let the survivor know you care, do what you can, then make a decision to participate or not, depending on your particular needs and circumstances.

My husband was abused by his father. He isn't ready to confront his father yet, and thinks it's okay for our kids to spend time with their grandfather. I don't like the idea. My husband is convinced his father won't abuse the kids, but I don't want to take any chances. How should we resolve this conflict?

In this situation, I have a definite opinion. Where children are concerned, it's always best to err on the side of caution. I have heard hundreds of stories from survivors who were certain they were the only victim, only to find out years later that their brothers and sisters, nieces, nephews, sons, daughters, and sometimes grandchildren had all been abused by the same perpetrator, one abuser systematically working his way through several generations of the same family. My grandfather started abusing me when he was seventy-one years old. Age alone is not a deterrent.

Survivors often believe that there was something particularly wrong with them that caused them to be abused. This erroneous sense of being responsible for the abuse can create a set of blinders for the survivor, who can't conceive of the fact that the abuser would abuse other children as well. Abusers sometimes tell their victims, "You're the only one." "You're special." "If you let me do this with you, I won't hurt your sister." Abusers lie. The compulsion to have sex with children is rarely a one time thing.

Seriously ask yourself: "Would I let my child bond with a suspected child molester if he wasn't related to me?" If you found out that the local scoutmaster had a history of sexually abusing children, would you keep sending your son to scouting? If your babysitter was found guilty of molestation, would you keep paying her to take care of your baby girl? Why should your child's grandfather be treated differently?

We've all been raised with the commandment "Honor thy father and thy mother." But when people sexually abuse their children, they give up their right to be treated with respect and honor in the family. At the moment the survivor's father abused him, he gave up all the normal rights and privileges that go along with being a parent, including his right to have a relationship with his grandchildren.

In workshops with survivors, whenever this topic comes up,

there are always several participants who are wavering in setting limits with their abusive parents. One survivor invariably says he feels guilty about depriving his children of a relationship with their grandparents. Invariably, there are several other survivors, all extremely vehement, who've made the tragic mistake of not stepping in, not saying no. They tell him to stop feeling guilty and to take action. One woman said:

> I didn't do anything. I was sure the abuse was over. I was grown up now. He wouldn't do it again. But he did. My stepfather got to all three of my kids and my nieces and nephews, too. And he was in bed this whole time, recovering from a heart attack.

I've heard survivors (and partners) say, "But I'm there every minute. I make sure he's never alone with the kids." Doesn't this survivor ever go to the bathroom? Doesn't he ever turn his back to wash the dishes or reach for a drink in the refrigerator? It only takes thirty seconds to abuse a child. That thirty seconds can dramatically alter that child's life. It's not worth the risk.

The bottom line is that it's your job to protect your kids. This is one place where the survivor's judgment may be off. His interests (taking his time preparing to confront) and the safety of your children may be in direct conflict. This is one circumstance where the survivor may need to push himself. The safety of your kids has to come first.

One partner told the following story:

> Sylvia needed to tell her brothers. She needed to tell one brother before she was ready because he has two kids. He was leaving his kids with Sylvia's father. She went down and told her brother and her sister-in-law. They were real cool about it. They said, "Oh, that must have been real hard for you." And Sylvia said, "Yeah. And I really think you need to be careful with your kids. I'm really concerned about them." And her brother just said, "Well, that might have happened then. But Dad won't do that now." And Sylvia said, "They do it. They keep doing it." But they didn't listen. They kept sending their kids over there. For

another year or so, Sylvia wrestled with calling the police. She called the police six months ago, and they opened a case. Of course they put it on the back burner, but at least she took a public stand. She'd like to push it further.

Another partner had to step in and be the limit-setter in his family. At first he had trouble trusting his instincts, but later he found the strength to hold firm:

I don't want her father in my house. I don't want him around my children. A couple of years ago we did go back to visit for a few days, and he had his hands all over my daughter, wanting to pick her up, wanting to kiss her, even when she was trying to push him away. My wife's sister and brother-in-law were there. We were going to go out to the movies and leave the kids at home with their grandparents. I felt incredibly uncomfortable even though they were all going to be asleep before we left. I felt horrible. My wife said it was okay. I was sitting in the movie with knots in my stomach, feeling really horrible, sure we'd come home and she'd be awake and hanging out with him. I couldn't believe my wife hadn't supported me in it. We came back, and sure enough, she was awake and hanging out with them. I don't think anything happened. But I felt betrayed by my wife in that situation. When she's with her parents she loses her adult status and her adult sensibilities. But we haven't gone back there since then. I've been stronger about it and she has too.

It's easy for me to be absolute in my opinion about setting limits with potential abusers in my family. It's harder to say no in reality. Your children may already have a long-established relationship with their grandparents before the abuse is uncovered. The survivor may not be ready to confront and doesn't want to explain why the children aren't with you when you visit. You're not ready to tell your children why they can't see Grandpa anymore. These are all very difficult issues, but they must be faced if you want to protect your children.

What you need to keep reminding yourself when you feel like

wavering and giving in is that abuse has consequences. Although you may be criticized or called cruel for "wrenching your grandchildren from their rightful grandparents," you will be doing the right thing. You will be teaching your children about what a healthy family does: It faces its mistakes and protects its members from harm.

Of course, there will be loss involved. You and your children will have to grieve the loss. Your children may be angry at you and blame you. But in the end, your children will learn a crucial lesson— that abuse is not okay and will not be tolerated in your family. You will have successfully broken the silence, and therefore, the cycle of abuse.

My wife was abused by her mother. We've decided not to let her see the kids anymore. What should we tell the children?

The truth. Children deserve accurate information about their families. That includes information about a child abuser in the family. It's not fair to give children a limited amount of information and then hope for the best. What kind of message does it give a child to say, "We're going over to Grandma's house. Don't let her hug you"?

Talking about abuse is a family issue. Everyone is involved; everyone needs to know. Information should be given to your children in a way that's age-appropriate. For a very young child, you could say something as simple as "Mommy's been crying and going to a lot of meetings at night because of something that happened to her when she was a little girl. She's taking care of herself so that she can be a better mommy to you." An older child can get more specific information. With programs about abuse prevention in the curriculum of many schools, you may have a natural opening to bring up the subject. It's okay to name names. Children don't need graphic details, but Grandma should not be protected. That's how abuse gets passed from generation to generation. (For two examples of parents talking to their children, see "Virginia's Story" on page 293 and "Jack's Story" on page 245.)

I recently saw the movie *The Music Box.* In it, a daughter takes on the defense of her immigrant father, who's been accused of Nazi war crimes. The man has been a devoted father and grandfather for forty years. His grandson adores him. Numerous scenes show what a beautiful relationship they have with each other. The daughter is certain her father has been wrongfully accused and successfully defends him. The case is dropped. But as the movie nears its conclusion, she gets undeniable proof that he was, in fact, a sadistic butcher, responsible for the torture, rape, and murder of numerous Jews and Gypsies. In the movie's climax, she confronts her father (who has just been teaching his delighted grandson to ride a horse). He denies everything. She pounds his chest and cries, "Why, Poppa? Why?" Then she pulls back, looks him in the eye, and says, "You'll never see your grandson again. You have no grandson."

After days of soul-searching and little sleep, she sends the damning photos she has uncovered to the prosecutor of the case, with a note explaining what she's found. The case is reopened, this time with absolute proof. The movie's final scene shows the daughter going out her front door, picking up the newspaper, looking at the photos of her father and the accompanying story, printed on page one, and then coming back indoors to her son. She has him set down his schoolbooks and sit down on the bench for a long talk. She's going to tell him the truth about his grandfather. Roll the credits. Fade out.

I found *The Music Box* powerful and provocative. It clearly showed the need to deny and the courage it takes to confront reality. The daughter was transformed (and almost torn apart) by the revelations about her father, but she was somehow able to integrate the horrible truth and move on. She didn't protect her father or her son from the truth. She was a strong role model for survivors and partners.

You and the survivor will have to find your own way of talking to your children, but make sure you do. If you don't, your children will most likely blame themselves for the disappearance of their grandparents (or for the survivor's grumpiness, withdrawal, anger, or sadness). You're trying to break the cycle of family silence. Talking honestly with your kids is a good way to begin.

Our daughter was abused by my wife's father. What can we do to help her?

When a child is abused, the most crucial thing is to stop the abuse and tend to the child. You can't undo the abuse that's already happened. Your son or daughter is living with the consequences. So are you. As parents, it's easy to get caught in feeling guilty for not having known, or to blame each other for having let the abuse go on. Remember that abuse is always the abuser's fault. It's a terrible tragedy that you don't see it or stop it, but there's nothing you can do about that now. What you can do is be good parents today. Let your son or daughter know you are sorry, that you should have seen and stopped the abuse. Tell your child, "No matter what you did, you weren't to blame."

Your child is a victim now, too. Don't assume she's resilient or that she can bounce back easily. The survivor is living proof that abuse festers underground. Find appropriate treatment for your child (preferably with peers who've also been abused). Get professional help so the injury can be resolved in childhood.[1]

As a family, you can opt to take action against the abuser (take him to court, sue for damages, confront him within the family) so your child has a chance to see the abuser punished. Your child should have the biggest say in any such action. Going to court is a big step. The justice meted out in our court system is rarely just, particularly in the realm of child sexual abuse. The decision to take legal action should not be made lightly. Make sure all of you understand the trade-offs involved, so that your decision is well-informed.[2]

When abuse is disclosed by adult children, the dynamics are similar. Your first concern should be with the survivor's needs, not with your own remorse, guilt, or grief. Don't waste time justifying what you did or didn't do. Don't push the survivor to forgive or absolve you of your guilt. Your adult children may be angry at you

---

[1] *The Mother's Book: How to Survive the Incest of Your Child* by Carolyn Byerly can be a valuable resource. See "For Parents" in the bibliography.

[2] For more on the controversy over how courts are handling child sex abuse cases, see *The Battle and the Backlash* by David Hechler. *By Silence Betrayed* by John Crewsdon, and *On Trial: America's Courts and Their Treatment of Sexually Abused Children* by Billie Wright Dziech and Judge Charles Shudson. See the "About Sexual Abuse" section of the bibliography.

for not protecting them; that's their right. Don't let their anger stop you from taking responsibility for your part and doing whatever you can to support their recovery.

Parents are often wracked with guilt when they find out that their children have been abused. They are paralyzed by shame; obsessed with "What if's" and Why didn't I's." Deal with these issues on your own. Put your guilt aside and take action: stop the abuse, confront the offender, protect your children, get them the help they need. In doing so, you will give your children something truly valuable: a model for facing the truth and healing wounds.

Focus on ways you can be a nurturing parent now. This is true whether your child is six, sixteen, or forty-six. Supporting your child in the present won't take away the fact that you didn't see or stop the abuse, but it can have a significant impact on the way abuse affects your children in the future. In actively supporting your child, you enhance her healing and make room for a healthier relationship between you.*

---

* An excellent book on improving relationships with adult children is *Making Peace with Your Adult Child* by Shauna Smith. See the bibliography for details.

Do survivors ever abuse their own children?

Although a majority of survivors become protective, empowering parents, some do go on to abuse their children or choose spouses who do. *If there is abuse going on in your home, it is imperative that you stop it and get help now.*

Families vary in terms of limit-setting, communication styles, strictness and leniency, styles of disciplining children. In one family, everybody yells. That's normal. In another, disagreements are discussed without ever raising a voice. In one family, parents are strict and the children are tightly controlled; in another, children are allowed more freedom. There are varying cultural and philosophical differences in the ways we raise our children. But there are certain behaviors that are abusive, no matter what. Here are some guidelines to help you determine whether you or the survivor have crossed that line and are abusing your children:

- **Physical abuse:** hitting, burning, slapping, pinching, whipping, biting, beating, or otherwise physically injuring a child, whether or not bruises, broken bones, or internal injuries result.
- **Emotional abuse:** belittling or humiliating a child; calling a child names; threatening to abandon or give a child away; attacking the child's self-esteem; lying to a child or manipulating the child's sense of reality.
- **Neglect:** failing to provide food, clothing, shelter, medical care, or adequate supervision.
- **Sexual abuse:** forcing, manipulating, or tricking a child into any kind of sexual contact. Participating in any sexual activity with a child is sexual abuse whether or not the child seems willing. Sexual abuse also includes (but is not limited to) forcing a child to watch sexual acts, making sexual comments to a child, taking sexual pictures of a child, and denying a child the right to privacy.

Part of being a good parent is being able to confront your own behavior or the behavior of your partner. *If you or the survivor are doing any of these things, you are abusing your children, and must stop. Seek help immediately.* Call Parent's Anonymous at 1-800-421-0353 or the National Child Abuse Hotline at 1-800-422-4453. If you think abuse is happening but you're not sure, call a parental stress hotline to talk about it. *Don't try to deal with this alone.* If you or the survivor haven't abused your children but are afraid that you might, get help now.

Once you call a public agency (or tell a therapist, doctor, teacher, or other professional), they are legally bound to investigate your situation. If they find abuse, they are mandated to file a report with child protective services. This can lead to involvement with social workers, police, and the criminal justice system, and may mean your children being temporarily removed from your home, but it can also mean getting the help you need.

Abusive parents have successfully stopped abusing their children. It is possible to confront abusive behavior and change; to find alternative ways of dealing with the stresses and frustration all parents experience. But in order to do so, you will need counseling and professional support. Don't hesitate in reaching out. *Protecting your children should be your number-one priority.*

My father was a violent alcoholic; my lover was sexually abused by both parents. We have terrible role models on both sides. We want to have children, but are afraid we are doomed to repeat our parents' mistakes. Is it really possible to be different?

Yes. It is possible to be different. Being abused as a child doesn't mean you are destined to abuse your own children, although this myth is propagated with great regularity. A recent *Parade Magazine* supplement in the Sunday paper featured the shocking headline WHAT IF THEY HAD LIVED?[1] It showed pictures of ten children who had been murdered by abusive parents. Inside, another headline screamed: "ABUSED CHILDREN WHO SURVIVE THEIR TORTURE ARE THE POTENTIAL RECRUITS FOR AN EVER-GROWING ARMY OF PREDATORY CRIMINALS." This kind of sensationalized journalism reinforces the idea that abused children inevitably become abusers.

While it's true that most abusers were abused as children, the opposite is *not* true. The majority of survivors *do not* go on to abuse children; the majority go on to become the protectors of children. If you and the survivor are willing to make a commitment to heal yourselves and learn healthy parenting skills, you will not be "destined" to abuse.

If you had poor or inadequate parenting yourself, and lack the proper instincts and skills to do the right thing with your children, you're in good company. You fit in with most of the other people trying to raise children. One survivor, a mother with sons aged nine and twenty, explains:

> When I was twelve I realized my parents were crazy, and that anything they did, I should do the opposite. I had my first son when I was nineteen. Whatever my gut inclination was with him, I questioned it. I asked myself, "Would my parents have done this? Is it sane or crazy?" Then I usually did the opposite.

---

[1] Andrew Vachss, "What if They Had Lived?" *Parade Magazine, Boston Sunday Globe,* June 3, 1990.

Parenting is a learned skill, not an innate talent. Like everyone else, you have to learn to be a good parent. Having been raised in a damaging environment, you know what you want to avoid. But it isn't enough to just hope you'll be different. Loving your child and doing the best you can are by themselves not sufficient to ensure good parenting. No one plans to be a bad parent, to act out a negative past. Repeated patterns of abuse happen when parents don't have support and haven't made a strong commitment to actively change.

The number-one rule of parenting, especially if you've come from a troubled family, is don't try to do it without help. Make the commitment to educate yourself about healthy boundaries, appropriate guidance, nurturing, building self-esteem in children, and other aspects of positive parenting.

Fortunately, there are many excellent resources now available for parents. There are books on child development, effective parenting, teaching self-esteem, healthy boundaries, and negotiating with children. (See "For Parents" in the Bibliography.) There are support groups for parents all over the country and centers that offer relief to stressed parents. You may have to do some searching, but you should be able to find resources in your local area. If not, start your own. Tack a note up at the local playground or at your pediatrician's office. There are parents who need support everywhere.

If you walk into parenting with your eyes open and a willingness to learn, it's possible to become an empowering, protective parent. And along the way, you'll probably gain some healing for yourself.

Mike and Julie have two children under the age of five. Julie was sexually abused by her father; having children has been a big part of her healing. As Mike explains, it's helped him, too:

> We make babies well and easily. Our daughter's birth was a powerful bonding for us. It was a healing time for me. It was the one time I saw Julie trust me totally, without any reservations. I'd never seen her so vulnerable and open and willing to accept me.
>
> Our second baby was born at home, too. Again it was a strengthening experience. But our son came out looking like Julie's father. It shocked her that he could look so much like him. She worried that she'd given birth to her

father again; she kept saying, "You can't be reincarnated before you're dead, can you?" As our son fills out, he looks less like him. We're both glad.

For Julie, it's been good having a boy: seeing a little boy, a little penis, seeing it as a nonthreatening thing; seeing she can love a boy as much as she loved a girl. She looks to our son as a healing force in her life. Every day she says things like, "I didn't know a boy could be so sweet, so cute, so nice." Until she had him, she thought every woman who professed to love a boy was actually faking it. Now she says, "Oh, those women really did love their kids. I know because I love this little guy."

It is possible to radically change family patterns from one generation to the next. No one has to repeat what was done to them as a child. When you face the truth about your own family and make the commitment to develop healthy parenting skills, you can gain the self-awareness, humility, insight, and resources necessary to break the cycle of abuse.

FINAL THOUGHTS

"All the reasons we got together were sick, but we've been able to turn them around."

"People who go through life without any problems seem kind of superficial to me now. This has deepened me as a person. It's forced me to really question a lot of things about life and human relationships. And any time you're forced to question a lot of things, and come up with your own answers, you become a stronger person with more depth."

Frankly, I'm not enjoying the current stage. I wonder what I have to look forward to. What will the survivor be like after therapy? What differences or changes will there be?

You actually have a lot to look forward to. Survivors who have actively faced their healing are some of the most lively, spunky, brave, funny, wonderful people I know. There's something about diving into the deepest pain of life and coming out whole, that leads us to enjoy each precious moment of life, because we know it's all we've got. Instead of responding to the pain of the past, survivors learn to appreciate the wild beauty of the present.

Before someone has dealt with his sexual abuse, he's likely to act from a lot of old self-protective programs developed in response to the abuse. These are often unconscious—the survivor isn't sure why he pulls away when someone gets close, has panic attacks, or needs absolute control over every detail of his life. But he—and you, by extension—is at the mercy of these ingrained patterns. As a survivor moves further along in his healing, he gains the freedom and ability to make choices that are not predetermined by the abuse. Instead of automatically responding in narrow, limited ways, his options broaden. The world opens up to something scary and brand-new. Instead of acting tough or responding like a perpetually scared victim, the survivor will be able to ask, "How do I want to handle this situation?" "What new skills can I use here?" "What kind of person do I want to be?" "What are the things I've always wanted to try?" As a partner, you will be part of this process of discovery. It's thrilling to watch someone you love see the world through new eyes.

The survivor's life will also stabilize. At the beginning of the healing process, obsession with sexual abuse is the norm. Everything is seen through abuse-colored glasses. Every man or woman walking a child on the street is a potential child molester; every problem in life is a direct result of the abuse. Pain and flashbacks lurk behind every corner. Nothing is simple or predictable. "Normal life" is out of the question.

As he heals, the survivor will experience increasing calm, greater stability, and more and more moments that are simply moments, not tainted or shadowed by abuse. There will be time between traumas.

And eventually, traumas will be the exception, not the rule. The survivor's life will become increasingly focused on living, rather than healing. Sexual abuse will gradually fade as his number-one concern. And as he reexperiences pleasure, relaxation, and laughter, so will you.

Your relationship will change, too. You will feel less like a caretaker and more like an equal partner. You will not have to be so careful about everything you do and say. The survivor will be able to pay more attention to your feelings and needs, and you will feel less like you're taking a back seat. As you both heal your childhood pain, the present, and your shared life in it, will take on increased importance.

Even your fights and conflicts will change. You'll stop feeling that the abuser is right there with you, involved in every fight or standoff. Your problems will have more to do with your own eccentricities and present-day needs. The impact of sexual abuse will no longer be the focal point of your growth together as a couple.

Sexually, your relationship should improve. Once the survivor has gone through the initial healing stages, he'll be able to actively choose and participate in sexual healing. Things may not be exactly the way you want them to be, but you'll sense movement and progress in your sexual life—you'll have a common goal, you'll work together, things will change over time.

When you're with a survivor who has done significant healing, you're with someone who has shown enormous stamina, vulnerability, and courage. If he's been able to weather this (and you have, too), the further challenges life brings will seem easy by comparison. If you survive a hurricane, a smaller squall seems pretty manageable.

Although there is no definitive end to healing, there is an end to the constant sense of struggle that accompanies the early stages of the healing process. When I talk to couples who've made it through the wrenching, chaotic early years, they talk not about the pain, but about their pride in what they've accomplished. When asked, they can talk about how hard things once were, but generally they're too busy getting on with their lives to spend much time dwelling on the past. I see in these couples a sense of confidence about their ability to face the future, both individually and together. "If we made it through that," they frequently say, "we can do anything."

PART II:
PARTNERS' STORIES

PARTNERS' STORIES:
An Introduction

In the course of writing this book, I talked to hundreds of partners and interviewed twenty-five in depth. The eight stories in this section have been chosen to represent a wide range of partners' experiences. You'll meet heterosexual men and women, lesbians, and gay men. You'll meet partners who have left relationships (or are thinking of leaving) as well as partners who are deeply committed. You'll meet men and women who are hopeful and positive and others who are struggling with life-threatening crises. It is my hope that you'll be able to identify with at least several of the men and women who have generously offered to share their stories with you.

These stories are written from the partner's point of view. Since this is primarily a book for partners, I chose not to interview couples. Although the survivors involved read and approved the stories, they weren't interviewed, and the stories don't represent their feelings, needs, or perspective with equal weight. I also didn't choose stories based on the diversity of survivor's experiences. As you read, you'll see there are no examples of abuse by mothers, brothers, strangers, and a host of other perpetrators. There are three survivors of cult abuse, and no examples of one-time sexual abuse or covert incest. This in no way minimizes the impact or importance of those experiences. It merely represents my limitations as an author needing to limit the number of pages in this book. I faced difficult choices; in the end I chose stories based on the diversity of the partners' experiences.

The stories are written in the first person; I tried to retain the unique flavor of each person's language and style of talking. The pieces were edited down from longer interviews and represent only a small portion of what each partner said. Each interview depicts only one moment in time: the day the interview took place. Often when I sent the interviews back, the partners and survivors said, "But so much has happened since then. We're not in that place anymore." Relationships aren't static; they're changing all the time. Like all of us, the people in these stories have continued to grow.

As you read through these stories, take your time. Give yourself a chance to digest each one. Let these men and women enter your life and your dreams; their words and actions will inspire you, sometimes when you least expect it. Having lived with these stories for many months, I frequently find myself having imaginary conversations with these partners in my head. I'll say, "Oh, yeah. Now I'm acting just like Scott and Jim when they were arguing in the car." Or I'll be struggling in my relationship and I'll ask myself, "How would Jack have handled this?" "Or I'll think, "Virginia and Keith worked it out. So can we." Let these stories live with you for awhile; you might be surprised by the results.

ABOUT NAMES

Except for Scott and Jim, everyone represented in these stories is using a pseudonym; identifying details have been changed in each story. Some of the partners and survivors chose to disguise their identities so they could protect their privacy; others wanted to use their real names, but couldn't for legal reasons. Unless the abuser was dead (as was the case with Jim), or had been convicted of sexual abuse in court, we risked a libel suit if we identified the abusers through the use of real names. I talked this over with the people who wanted to use their own names, and they agreed that their stories were important enough to compromise and use pseudonyms. This is yet another case where the law protects the abusers, instead of the abused. Like many of the laws regarding child sexual abuse, it, too, must be changed.

JACK'S STORY:
Recovering Together

Jack and his wife, Valerie, are both thirty-six years old. They've been married for twelve years and have three children, aged five, eight and ten.

I'm the oldest of two boys. My dad dealt with problems through silence and rage; my mom used withdrawal and drinking. I learned those ways pretty well. Early on, I learned emotions were dangerous. They caused trouble. I couldn't ever show what I felt.

I met Valerie in 1969. We were fifteen when we started dating. We moved apart, but got back together at twenty-one. We married two years later.

When she was fifteen, Valerie told me about the abuse, but said it didn't affect her. The effects didn't surface until our son was born, about a year after we married. Our sex life took a nosedive. There was a total lack of desire on Valerie's part. According to her, it always had something to do with me. I accepted it on the surface, but raged on the inside.

For the first eight years after our son was born, until two years ago, things deteriorated in a more or less steady way. I'd initiate sex and she'd say, "No, no, no, no," until at one point I stopped asking. The initiation of sex was taken out of my hands for a reason I didn't understand. The reasons she said no ranged from, "You drink and you come to bed smelling like beer and alcohol" to "Your eyebrows are too bushy. I can't have sex tonight."

We got into this cycle. The sex thing would trigger resentment in me. I'd get angry, withdraw, and then lash out. Then we'd have sex and things would be okay for a while. Two or three months later, the same cycle would repeat. And each time, the trough would get deeper. It became intolerable. I started drinking more and more. I was in my own downward spiral with alcohol, all the time denying that anything was wrong with me. I blamed everything on her because she couldn't have sex.

Things finally came to a head. One day, after she turned me down again, I lay there in total defeat and said, "I think what your grandfather did to you is having a huge effect on your life. More than you or I want to admit. This just isn't right. For ten years, we haven't been able to have the sex life we want." And she said, "Okay, I'll look into it." She made an appointment with a counselor. The whole thing started right there.

About that time we took a vacation to Mexico with a couple of friends. We told them we were starting marriage counseling. We told them why. The man started making some old hackneyed jokes that indicated how uncomfortable he was with the whole thing, and he and Valerie really got into it. When we got back to our room, she came unglued. She flipped out into this uncontrollable crying. She kept sobbing, "What's wrong with me? What's wrong with me?" She was lost in a bottomless pit of hopelessness.

I felt helpless. I held her. I tried to say some reassuring words. But I was really blown away by the depth of her despair and how bleak she sounded. It was scary. I'd never seen anyone cry uncontrollably before. When I look back now, I see it was a sign of the damage that had been done. She was beginning to realize just how hurt she'd been. And this was after only one counseling session.

STARTING MY RECOVERY

My recovery from alcoholism was definitely triggered by her being a survivor. All the issues came together. I was rejected a lot for sex because I smelled like booze. Her grandfather drank. One day, our counselor said to me, "You probably won't get much better unless you quit drinking." I guess I was ready to hear it. I got heavily involved in AA. For the first time, I was looking inside myself without a lot of cynicism or self-loathing. I started feeling better about myself. I started some counseling on my own, looking at issues in my own family.

A lot of my intense reactions to Valerie's abuse issues have to do with my own pain. One area that's really shown up is around the initiation of sex. If I initiate sex the wrong way with Valerie, I'm not just risking a bad mood, I'm risking a terrible emotional experience for her. The times I initiated sex and was rejected even when I thought I did everything right ("Your nose hair's too long." "You didn't shave"), I withdrew right away. Later I'd intensify my withdrawal and lash out with hurtful words. In the depths of this real self-pitying resentfulness, I'd feel like I hated her. And I don't hate Valerie. I'd have to stop and say, "Where's this coming from?" And I knew it was coming from this little kid inside of me who'd been rejected.

DEALING WITH HER PAIN

She's gone through severe identity crises, combined with depression and hopelessness. I still feel overwhelmed and incapable of dealing with a lot of it, partly because of how we interact. Words have been critical in our relationship. I have felt at times, by using the wrong word with Valerie—the wrong word about sex or the wrong word in describing a person—that she's completely devastated and can't relate to me anymore.

Sometimes she asks questions I can't answer. She'll say, "Do you think I have multiple personalities?" And right away I have this committee inside my head that says, "Make sure you choose the right word." What does she need to hear from me when she's in crisis and asking that question? Out of self-defense, I often say things like, "I don't know. I'm not a psychiatrist. I can't answer that." If I'm in a better place, I listen and probe a little bit.

One of the things Valerie has learned is to take care of the little kid in her. Her little kid is really scared and needy. At first when she came out, I was really confused. It's frustrating to have an adult act like a child. I didn't understand why she couldn't just cope. I'd think, "C'mon, snap out of it. You're a big kid. I know it's bad, but you don't have to be doing this right now. Snap out of it." That's how I reacted early on. As I move through my own recovery, I'm more able to be there for her. But it still feels weird. My image of myself with Valerie is as a husband and a lover. I don't feel comfortable in the parental role with a real needy kid. She's had to turn to her counselor for that a lot.

Another thing that's been hard for me to deal with is the dissociation. It still happens quite a bit. There are many variations of it. The intense kind is when I have to come rescue her. I'd call from work and she'd be overwhelmed. I'd have to pick her up and drive her somewhere. Or I'd have to take the kids because she couldn't cope.

The second kind of dissociation feels like I'm split off from her. I'll tell her, "You're showing contempt for me right now. You haven't got any idea who I am. There's no emotional tie between us. You've forgotten I'm a person who matters." She used to deny it. Now she says, "Yeah, I'm seeing bad Jack." This used to really confuse me. How could I be Mr. Wonderful All-American one day and not be able to tie my shoes right the next? She'd be totally detached from me and the kids.

The third kind of dissociation is when she has flashbacks. She'll say, "Right now, I'm having a flashback." A significant number of them come before, during, and after sex. Others come up after therapy or in dreams. The ones before, during, and after sex are really hard. They wreck things. She'll be sobbing after she has an orgasm, struggling against a memory that's pounding at the door. At first when she said, "I want you out of this bed," I felt resentful and hurt. Now I say, "What can I do? How can I be here for you?" Then I try to do whatever she asks for. It's just what's needed.

I've had to reach a certain level of self-acceptance and self-esteem or I'd never be able to deal with this. There's so much rejection, hurt, and pushing away. At first it was devastating. It was rejection after rejection. Knowing what I know about my family now, I realize that's a life-and-death issue for me. That's why this intensity of feelings would come up.

Sometimes I've gotten angry. Not at her, but at this phantom wrecking our lives. We're in a place now we've never been before. We're more whole, but because of the sexual abuse, the sexual part of our lives has been unable to heal as fast as the other parts of our relationship. That's really frustrating. Sexuality is still so loaded. It's tough. Rules of silence can still prevail. I resent that about our recovery together. It's an area in which we could really grow, and it's lagging behind. I wish it was happening faster.

WE ALMOST SPLIT UP

Six months ago, about eighteen months into recovery, we almost split up. It was too much. I was at a place where it was important for me to have some hope about having a normal sex life. And Valerie was at a place where she couldn't see how that would ever be possible. She couldn't make any commitment to that being possible. And I couldn't accept that. As I've recovered, I've realized I deserve to have the things in life I want. And one thing that's important to me is a healthy sex life.

I got to the point where I said, "This is really hard for me. I need a sex life where I can explore. I want to do it with you, but you say you can't, that you'll probably never be able to. I need some hope or I'm out of here." I was assertive and Valerie felt like a victim. The situation seemed hopeless. We started talking about who was going to move out, who was going to arrange day-care. We didn't get to the financial details, but we were close. Our differences seemed irreconcilable.

When I thought about us splitting up, I got terribly frightened. As we inched closer, I started to feel the loss. I was poised on the brink of this devastating loss, and it was just a foreshadowing of what was to come. It was monumental. I thought about the impact it would have on the kids. I had real strong feelings about that, and I was able to pay attention to them. Two years ago I couldn't have done that. It made us stay together.

Coming up to this brink brought me back to something our counselor said when we first went to counseling. He said, "You have to make a commitment." And I said, "Yeah, I'm committed, definitely." And in all honesty, what I meant was, "Yeah, I'll show up here every week." That was about it. What he was talking about was, "When you get to this place, when you get to this wall, you find a way over or around, but you don't turn around and walk away from it. You find a way through it."

For me, that's been very painful because it involves a number of things I've spent my life avoiding—compromise, deep self-evaluation, being responsible for my actions. It requires assertiveness and initiative, which means being in touch with my feelings enough to know what the hell I want. It means finding a way to get my needs met within this relationship.

I thought a lot about commitment and it took on a new meaning for me, a deeper meaning, not just showing up but, "Here we are. This is tough. Let's look it in the face and try to get through it somehow." And we did. I felt a new depth of commitment to my family.

DEALING WITH HER FAMILY

I have revenge fantasies all the time. I've written a few pages of a short story based on her last visit to her grandfather. He was getting oxygen. He was incontinent. His lifetime of bad habits had caught up to him. He was pitiful. I've never had any empathy or sympathy for him. That whole trip I kept thinking about how easy it would be to just undo his oxygen.

Another fantasy I had goes like this: He's in the hospital. He's on his deathbed. All the relatives are crowded around doing their thing. "Goodbye. You had a good life." And I walk up to him and say, "You lousy old fucker. I know what you did. I'm glad to see you go," and then I pull out a gun and shoot him in front of everyone. The idea of humiliating him in front of the family is really powerful.

I'm sorry now I never confronted him. It feels like a rite of passage I missed. But this was years before my own recovery and I didn't have the courage or strength. In fact, when Valerie first came to me and said she wanted to confront her family, I was a codependent baby. I said, "Don't upset the apple cart. Bad things will happen if you do this." I have a fear of people being mad at me. It's the kid in me: "I don't care what he did. I want to be liked." That's life and death for me, at least it used to be. As my recovery has progressed, I've been more supportive of her feelings about her family. I let her decide what's comfortable for her.

The biggest issue for us in terms of her family has been her brother. Five years ago, he was arrested and convicted of child molesting and spent time in jail for it. Valerie and I talked a few times about if and how our kids should interact with him. Valerie wanted to keep the kids away from him. I didn't back her up. Instead of saying, "No, I don't think the kids should see Bob either," I'd say, "Gee, I don't know. What do you want to do? If we do tell Bob he can't see the kids, there'll be hell to pay in the family. But of course, it's your decision." Really wimpy, unhelpful crap. I recognize that now. I focused on everyone else's feelings except my family's well-being. Valerie would get frustrated and drop it. It was too upsetting.

As my recovery progressed, it became crystal clear to me where the priorities were. If she hadn't talked to Bob and set a limit this Christmas, I would have. We finally were of one mind in this. There was no question about it. A couple of months before the annual Christmas get-together, she called him and asked him about his recovery and his desires. She learned he still has sexual desires for boys and that when his probation is up, if a situation arises, he would avail himself of it. Because of our kids, we had to make a judgment. Valerie called him and said, "We're not going to see you this Christmas. You're not going to see our kids." He said, "You're overreacting. It's a big mistake." Her mother said the same thing. Her younger brother was more supportive.

The weird thing is there had still been so much silence that hardly anyone in the family knew he'd been to jail for molesting kids. We told everybody. It upset things. "Why does everyone have to know? It's over. Why are you doing this?" We said, "When some-one has Bob's problem, people with kids need to know about it. We just can't keep the silence anymore. It's not healthy. We can't pre-tend this didn't happen."

We've also been very forthright and open with our kids. They know why Mom sometimes can't cope and has to go into her room and write for a few hours. Or why she can't take a lot of noise. The two oldest know who did it. They don't know specifically what he did, but they know he touched her sexually and made her touch him in a way that was inappropriate. Our five-year-old just knows who it was and that he did bad things to Mom, and that Mom's mad about it.

The older kids asked a bunch of questions at first. Then they'd seem to forget it. A month later, they'd ask another question. That's how they've handled the revelations of the last two years. When I sat them down and told them I was alcoholic, they were pretty interested for about ten minutes, then it was, "What's on TV?" A month later they asked, "Can I come to a meeting sometime?" or "What do you talk about at those meetings?" We're always honest and open with them in terms they can understand.

I have seen the price Valerie is paying for what happened to her in her family. It's clear to me now that what we do with our kids is going to show up for them later in their lives. It's been a real important lesson on priorities. I try to be there for our kids, not just for traumas and tragedies but for everyday stuff, to be connected to them. I'm far from perfect at it, but I'm aware of it.

RECOVERING TOGETHER

Between the two of us with our recovery issues, it's been trigger city. It's not very safe. Sometimes she's in a place where she's doing well and I'm a mess. Times like that, we don't get along very well. We get into dueling recovery—basically, who's less fucked up. We get into spitting contests about who's doing better. "I'm not happy with your recovery," or "I'm sick of this behavior and you're still not doing anything about it."

The worst thing about recovery is there's no covering up. There's no need for her to pretend that sex was great and that she didn't have these feelings. There's no need for me to say, "No, I'm not mad about it."

I've learned to handle the overt rejection. Don't get me wrong. I'm not a pro at it. I don't welcome it. It's not the highlight of my day when it happens. But when it happens, I don't die over it. I don't drink over it. I don't rage over it. I can handle it now.

I've learned that I can't deny her the right to have whatever feelings she's having just because they're uncomfortable for me; that I don't have control over her emotions. I have to let her walk through her own shit and learn what she can from it. That's the only way she's going to get better.

I used to think that nurturing and supporting meant trying to steer her away from this terrible stuff into "Things are okay. You're wonderful. You'll be okay," but it isn't. Nurturing is a combination of empathy and acceptance that comes from listening and not trying to deny or minimize her feelings. And being there in the way she finds comforting in the moment. Now I say to her, "How can I be here for you? What do you think would help right now? Do you want me to take the kids?" I try to give her a sense that no matter what she's feeling, I'm not going to freak out about it. I may freak out about it later, but in the moment, I'm not going to jump up and run away. Whatever she needs, if I can give it, I will.

I'm still trying to learn to balance my needs with hers. For instance, I've had to set limits on my own time. Valerie likes to talk about incest a lot. At times it seems like an obsession. Sometimes, I don't want to listen. I used to react by either listening with one ear or doing some real passive-aggressive stuff—fidgeting, moving around, turning the radio up a little louder. Now I say, "I don't want to listen to this right now. This isn't a good time for me. Can you call someone else?"

The thing that's given me hope through all this is the work Valerie has put in, the countless hours she's put in working on her issues, the growth she's had. Little by little, she's let go of the control she's needed. She has a lot more acceptance, tolerance, and willingness to deal with problems. She takes responsibility for her actions and feelings now. I take responsibility for my part. That's given us both a lot of hope.

One of the best things about being in recovery together is finding new common ground. An example is prayer. That's part of what I got into in AA. Meditation and self-reflection is very much part of the program. Religion was never anything Valerie or I shared. When she got into recovery, we were able to talk about prayer and share that with one another. We have a free flow of honest, open feelings and emotions with each other without a lot of the old baggage that used to crowd our interactions.

We're on a road of personal and spiritual growth. We're on it together, but separately. I've gotten there from my addiction to alcohol and Valerie from her abuse, but we're both on the same road. I don't know where it's going to lead us, but I know it's going to be good.

MARISE'S STORY:
"She Works Really Hard and So Do I"

Marise grew up in "a pretty nice home," the fifth of seven children. She and her partner, Jo, have been together for six years. Jo was abused by her brother and her father, and has been dealing with the memories for the last two years.

We just celebrated our sixth anniversary. We were together for four and a half years before she had any memories. And we had a lot of conflict during that period. We had solid communication about every other area, but when it came to sexuality, a wall went up. There was a lot of judgment from her because I liked sex a lot and she didn't. We would try to talk about it. She would get to a point where she would say, "Well, maybe it's me." But she would never go beyond that. And in every other aspect of our relationship, she'd always go to a deeper level to discover the cause.

She started getting memories two years ago. At first I felt frightened. I was afraid she was going to leave me. My only other knowledge of a survivor was a woman who had a really hard time, and then when she started feeling a little better, she left her lover and found someone new. I was afraid Jo would do that to me. So I worried a lot that we wouldn't make it. Instead, we've made our changes together. Since her memories, that wall isn't there anymore. We always go that extra level in our communication now. There's been real growth.

There was a time when I was afraid she was going to shut me out. And there was a time when she really considered it. She went through a period when she thought, "I could get out of this relationship and go through this alone." But she decided not to do that. She made a commitment to include me in her life, even though there are times she really wants to be alone. She has to deal with the fact that I am her partner. She can't run away from that. Even at her lowest, I get to be there too. I'm not ever completely cut out. She needs to be alone sometimes, and that's okay, but there's a kind of shutting out that doesn't happen. She made a commitment to include me in her life. She can't just take me when she wants me and push me away when she doesn't. I get to be a whole person. I get to be present. I don't feel invisible. When I feel bad, I get to have my feelings. She gives me the support to be myself.

When she first started dealing with the abuse, my response was to never tell her when I felt bad, because her problem was so much worse than mine. Finally, I started to be more honest with her. I started sharing my feelings more. It was a relief for her to have someone else's problems to think about. She liked knowing she could be there for me, that she wasn't always taking, but that she could also give. I had been holding back, and when I finally started opening up more, it ended up being helpful for her.

I had come to the conclusion that I'd rather be alone than be in a bad relationship. The good times are so good with her, it's helped me through the hard times. I've never really doubted being with her.

I'M A PASSIONATE PERSON

We had struggles around her not wanting sex as much as I did, and then it became even less. But the quality when she's there is so much better now. During the first four years of our relationship there were times she felt so guilty for not being sexual that she'd make love, but she wouldn't really be there—she'd have this out-of-body experience. Now when she wants to be sexual, she's really present. It's so much better than all the times she was sort of there.

In the beginning, I was rejected so often that I started repressing my sexuality. It was too painful for me to feel sexual when she didn't. Sex became associated with unpleasantness. And now it's not.

I had to look at the ways I let my self-esteem depend on whether or not she felt sexual. I was putting sexuality outside of myself, and I've had to learn to separate her sexuality from mine.

Our mutual goal is to each be true to our own sexuality. She wants to heal from the wounds and the pain. She's striving to be more open. My goal is to be true to myself. If I'm feeling sexual, it's okay. I'm a person who can feel sexual about anything. The way wind blows against my skin.

I've learned that it's okay to be a passionate person. That scared Jo a lot at first. She associated passion with being out of control. Not just sexual passion, but passion in life. At first, I was scared to let my passion out—passionate anger, passionate joy, passion over whatever I was doing. I tried to tone everything down for her. But being true to that passion inside me is what makes me alive, and I realized I couldn't live without it.

It's nice reclaiming it. I'm trying to acknowledge when I'm sexual and not to try to keep it secret, just to say it, not to expect anything back from her. I need to validate, "This is who I am and this is how I feel right now. I feel really sexy." She's been able to acknowledge my sexuality as a good thing. She's actually said she envies the free feeling I have about sex.

There are times I still get frustrated, but I don't get to that point where I'm pulling my hair out anymore. She's able to be sexual with me on a more regular basis. And I can be alone and masturbate and feel good about it.

WHY IT'S BEEN WORTH IT

I'm amazed by our communication. It's something I treasure. I didn't grow up with it and it's important to me. The first four years we built a sold basis in communication. It just keeps expanding.

My work life has changed. This is the first time in my life I have a job that challenges me. I'm growing at work. I'm getting paid well. I've never had that before. And I feel like this job is a direct result of our work together. My job requires communication skills I've developed for the relationship.

She has let go of so much control. That's been one of the best parts of the process. Jo was a major control freak. We would do these projects together. One time I got paint on the paintbrush handle and she flipped out. I put the brush down and said, "That's it." She's so much more relaxed that now it's enjoyable to do something like that together.

Jo's process has spurred my own growth over and over again. I'm more confident about facing challenges. My own personal growth has deepened. I've looked at things from my past that have controlled me all my life. I didn't even know they were controlling me. My religious background. My family. It's been a wonderful experience in that way.

Overall, I'd say our process parallels each other's. She works really, really hard and so do I. I've made a commitment to stick it out with her and to go through it together. I feel very committed.

NOAH'S STORY:
Crisis and Cult Abuse

Noah is a twenty-one-year-old actor. He and Jade, twenty-four, have been together for four and a half years, married for four. Jade was sexually abused by her father and also in a satanic cult. They have a three-year-old daughter, Gracie.

I always thought my childhood was perfect. I'm discovering now that it wasn't. My parents weren't abusive; it was all very quiet stuff. I was given anything I wanted: money was the main way my parents showed love. At twelve, they sent me to boarding school. I left school at fifteen and worked for a year. Then I went to acting school. That's where I met Jade.

It was strange the way we came together. It was so improbable. We're so different. I'm slow. She's a fireball. She's older than I am. She had so much more experience. She'd already been to acting school.

We had a bit of a friendship at first. Gradually, things fell together. By March, we were living together. We fought all the time, about everything. I was hanging on, "Don't leave me." And she was saying, "I'm leaving now." We still do some of that, four and a half years later, but not as much.

She was my first sexual partner. We didn't make love until we'd been living together for four months. It strengthened us to wait. I had so much anxiety around sex. I was terrified and scared. She was, too. It wasn't as obvious then. She was very numb.

We were just kids. We didn't know what we were doing. We talked about the possibility of her getting pregnant, and then, she did. At first she didn't want me around, but we stuck it out together.

After Gracie was born, Jade started having severe anxiety, terror, and nightmares. She couldn't sleep. Things would trigger her and she'd go into a rage. Things were exploding everywhere. She started having memories. We knew she'd come from a violent home, but not that she'd been sexually abused. She felt disbelief and terror. She'd say, "I know he hit me, but not this." Then she got into an incest survivors' group. It was all very quick.

How did I respond? As well as I could without knowing much. I'd never heard of sexual abuse, I didn't even know it happened, but the whole thing made sense to me. I'd heard so much about the violent abuse in her family, I wasn't surprised. I stood by her as best I could. I tried to validate her. I'd say, "From what I know of your family, this is very possible."

Back then I wasn't working. I was home most of the time. Our baby wasn't in day-care. Basically we were stuck together a lot of the time. Gracie was less than a year old. That was the heavy part. It wasn't just about being with Jade. When she's going through stuff and the baby is there, what do I do? Jade can dissociate or get scared. She's had panic attacks where she needs to go to the hospital. What do I do? I can't leave Gracie; it's not good for her to see this. But I can't leave Jade either; I'm scared she's going to hurt herself. Sometimes I have to leave the house with Gracie, and Jade has to call someone else. There's nothing else I can do.

I've had to take care of everything: make sure the money is coming in; take care of Gracie, take care of Jade; cook, clean. I switch on automatic. I don't think or feel much. I say, "This is what has to be done. Let's just do it."

Sometimes I think, "It's unfair. Why do I have to do all this?" But I don't usually let myself think about that. When that feeling comes up, I turn it towards her Dad. He's the one that did this.

What's not fair, not just for me but for all of us, is the life we have to live. It's far from a regular life. It's not like I go to work and make the money. We're totally broke. We're on welfare. I work a few days a week. We've barely been able to make the rent and pay for food. It's not because we're not willing to work. It's because her father abused her. That's what gets to me. We have to suffer, all of us as a family, because of that.

CULT ABUSE

Jade is still in crisis. In fact, things have gotten worse. She's remembered being ritually abused in a Satanic cult. She has multiple personalities. She's been in the hospital. Looking back now, the sexual abuse was pretty easy by comparison. Don't get me wrong— it was awful. But there's a lot of information about sexual abuse. There's a lot less about ritual abuse. Multiple personalities, there's almost nothing. So we're dealing with a lot less resources.

I suppose she's always had different personalities. It's not clear-cut: "This is a personality and this is a personality." It's more subtle than that. Mostly she's got a lot of little kids who want special things to eat. There's one kid who wants special cookies. I've been going out to buy special cookies for years. Looking back, it's happened since we've been together. It's more distinct now, but it's always been like this. We just didn't know what it was.

When the other people come out, I have to remind myself that this is someone else. That's not always easy for me to remember. We've made love when she's in one of her kids, and it's like the abuse all over again for her. It's not that I'm trying to abuse her, but the fact is, she *is* a kid. She's got a very mad little kid in there that breaks plates, breaks cups, throws things all over the house, scratches me, tries to hit me. I have to remind myself that this is a mad, hurt kid. I don't fight with her; I try and find a way to be on her side.

Things change all the time. One minute she trusts me, and the next she doesn't. It doesn't have much to do with me. Everything can be fine and five minutes later, things explode and the rest of the day is awful. That's the life we live.

DEALING WITH MEMORIES

When she has memories, I hold her. I remind her I'm there. I tell her she's safe, that she's okay. I remind her to breathe and try to get her to tell me what she's seeing. Often she won't. She'll scream or curl up and forget what she remembered. So I ask what's happening and write it down for her.

I am a bit in the dark about what's going on these days. When she was dealing with just the sexual abuse, she talked about it all the time. I'd know what was going on. But with the ritual abuse, she doesn't talk about it much because it sends her into a panic. She was brainwashed. She got electric shocks. And while she got electric shocks she was told if she ever talked about it, she would die. It's physical. She gets pains in specific areas where electrodes were— her chest and her abdomen—if she gets close to talking. She liter- ally feels like she's going to die if she talks about it. So it's difficult for me to get a lot of information. Most of the information I've gotten is through reading, going to workshops, or going through memories with her.

The ritual abuse memories are a lot more intense to go through. Linked to the memories is a lot of body pain, panic attacks, and screaming. She often hyperventilates; her pulse goes up to 130. The first thing I do is remind her to breathe. When she has calmed down a little, there are two options—either try and put it away and not go through it, which may be more appropriate to the situation, or go into it. I tell her, "As long as you're running, the fear and terror will be greater. If you turn around and face it, it can't hurt you. You have the power. You're the one who is chasing it." I say to her, "The sooner you go to the bottom of the pit, the sooner you're going to get out. The sooner we go down deep in there, the sooner we're going to get out, so let's just do it."

THERE'S SUCH A DEEP BOND BETWEEN ME AND MY PARTNER

There's such a deep bond between me and my partner. I feel like this is one of the reasons I'm here this time around. This is a healing process for me, too. Sometimes it feels like I'm just helping Jade, but I have learned so much going through this with her. I'm giving love and support to her, but it feels like I'm giving it to myself at the same time. I can't even really put it into words. From the very beginning when she first started going through memories, I had this feeling, "This is why I'm here."

Sometimes she feels happy. Sometimes she feels good. She's not stopping or giving in. She hasn't killed herself and she's still dealing with all of this. That's very hopeful. A lot of ritual survivors never make it. Children die. She made it through the abuse, and now, she's making it through the memories. She's going to make it. One day our life will be different.

Leaving isn't an option for me. I could say, "I don't deserve this," but neither does she. I want to help Jade go through this, but I also don't want it to happen to anyone else.

I came from a family where everything was hunky-dory and I married someone who was ritually abused. It has opened my eyes to what really goes on in the world. And I want it to stop. There's a crusade against abuse and I feel like I'm part of it. I want to commit a good chunk of my life to helping people going through ritual abuse and sexual abuse, to fighting it.

WHAT ABOUT MY NEEDS?

I can't really explain why I do this. It's a very good question, but I can't answer it. Sometimes I get lonely and depressed. Not simply because of what's happening with Jade, but because it affects everything in our lives. At this point I'm ready to get back into acting. I need to do something I love that's going to make us money. I need to audition, yet I don't see how I'm going to be able to do that. But I have to do it or I won't stay sane. I'll be so depressed I won't be any good to anybody. But if I do get work, what kind of commitment can I make to it?

I would love a simple life where we go out once a week and have a good time or just go away for a weekend. I'd like us to have a courtship. That's something we never had. Some escaping together. Some fun, light, exotic romance. We're both actors. I'd love it if we worked together someday. But our life isn't like that. We fight a lot. We don't sleep much. There are literally times we sleep an average of four hours a night, a mixture of having a baby and memories. And that can happen for months at a time. We're usually completely exhausted.

I wish sometimes I could be taken care of. But I don't feel like there's room for me to fall apart. If Jade's dissociating, dinner needs to be cooked, Gracie's screaming because she's hungry, the phone is ringing, we have no money and hardly any food, what happens if I fall apart? What the hell is going to happen? Maybe Jade would come back and take care of things. But I don't think of that. I'm a caretaker. I just flip on automatic and put on dinner and take care of the two of them. It's easier to do that than to risk anything else.

I'm a control freak. I keep telling Jade what she needs to do to take care of herself. And I think I should be perfect. Sometimes I say, "No, I can't," but very rarely. There's still a part of me that believes I have to take care of Jade to deserve her. So I put my needs aside, but that's not good for any of us. If I can't have something for myself, I'm not able to be present as a partner or a parent. Recently, we've gotten Gracie into a day-care situation we like. We get a break from parenting and Gracie gets to play with other kids. We've also made an agreement that there are certain things I have to do to take care of myself.

Last week I went for a massage. I've started playing squash every week; it's a great way to get out my frustrations. And I've gotten into therapy myself. I'm trying to turn the focus onto me.

But I still use Jade as a way to hide from myself. It's easy to blame everything on her because she's going through so much. Her pain is always greater. My problems are never as dramatic. I use what Jade's going through to hide from my own fears, my depression, sadness, and anger. I'm in the perfect circumstance to do that. Sometimes I try to make it look like she's doing something wrong when really it's something in me. For instance, I have a lot of shame about sex. When she approaches me sexually, instead of saying, "Oh God, this is terrifying," and acknowledging what's going on for me, I act cold and look at her like, "What's the matter with you?"

I actually think I'm the one who's responsible for the problems we have with sex. I feel more relieved when we don't have sex. Sometimes we have sex and it's wonderful, but it's certainly not the core of our relationship. Far from it. Very far from it.

I have a huge amount of work to do on myself. I've grown a lot, like I've said, and I've healed a lot, but I still have a huge amount to do that has nothing to do with Jade, but with myself. I'm starting to realize that I wasn't born with all this shame. Something must have happened for me to have all this shame about sex. The joke between us is, "When you're done with this, I'm probably going to go through it." Maybe I'm a survivor, too. I just don't want to know yet.

Sometimes we have the feeling that nothing is changing. But like a tree or like a bush during the winter, it's all undergrowth. We have a friend who had this bush that wasn't growing, so she uprooted it. It was a rosebush and it had grown thousands and thousands of roots. And in the springtime, she put it back in the soil and it just went crazy and sprouted everywhere. It's the same with this. Often Jade just feels so impatient and says, "Nothing is changing." But everyday something *is* happening. It *is* changing. Sometimes a little bud comes out and you can see it.

It's a long process. It takes years. She had her first sexual abuse memories two years ago; ritual abuse memories for about a year. She's moving very quickly. That makes me move very quickly. It seems very fast to me. I mean, I'm only twenty-one. Most twenty-one-year-olds I know are either still in school or hanging out at the mall. Having a baby and then dealing with the abuse has made me zoom light-years ahead of what I would have done otherwise. There's so much I have learned. I'm looking at the world through totally different eyes since I've gone through this. I care about people a lot more. I'm a lot more aware. I've grown up very fast. I wouldn't be who I am now if I hadn't gone through this with Jade. I'd just be a twenty-one-year-old kid without much to say.

ERIC'S STORY:
The Support of Others

Eric, forty-one, is a general contractor. His wife, Sarah, thirty-six, was sexually abused by her father. Married for six years, they have three children between them. The older two, eleven and nine, are from Sarah's first marriage. Their youngest is three and a half.

I was raised by my mother. My father died before I was five and my mother didn't remarry until I was an adult. I didn't have any brothers or sisters. It was a mom-son kind of thing.

My mom always was working to support us, but there was always a message that I was the man in the family; there to fix things and help take care of things. Life was tough for her and I got the message to be a good boy and not to give her any problems. I always got a lot of strokes for that as a kid, "You're such a nice boy, Ricky."

There were no strong male figures in my childhood. I never had a role model for what a husband or father, an adult male should be. Because of that, my first year of marriage, before the incest even came up, was a lot for me to handle. I went from living alone for ten years to suddenly having a wife and two stepkids overnight. It was a huge responsibility. I was scared shitless. I took it all very seriously, maybe too seriously. I felt I had to do everything right. I had to do this father thing right. I had to do this husband thing right. But I didn't know how to do either. I had no models.

ERIC'S STORY: THE SUPPORT OF OTHERS

About a year after we got married, Sarah first discovered the incest. She had been showing signs of something being drastically wrong all through her growing-up years. She was in and out of therapy as a teenager. The abuse never came up. Not much was known about incest at that time. We went to some premarital counseling. Nothing came up about the incest.

She had what she called "funny dreams and strange thoughts." She was pursuing that in therapy when we met. Throughout the day she kept getting these images. They were eating up a lot of her energy. She started having dreams and flashbacks she couldn't explain. Finally, she just realized it one day. It became clear to her in a therapy session what these memories were. Our lives changed dramatically from that day on.

I remember the day very clearly. She came home and was sitting at the table. I was at the kitchen counter and she told me. I went blank. It didn't sink in at first. I didn't have any understanding of the effect the incest had on Sarah. I feel bad about that now, but I didn't understand the magnitude of this; how brutal and devastating it could be. I really played it down.

From that day on, everything changed. It was like a hurricane going on around me. Sarah got obsessed with thoughts about the incest. I lost her as a wife and as a mother. All her waking and sleeping hours were taken up with this issue. There were days I'd come home from work and I wouldn't know where Sarah would be: if she'd be upstairs on the bed crying, where she'd been for the last four hours, or if she'd be downstairs fixing dinner, or if she'd just be gone.

I didn't know day-to-day if Sarah would be able to cope. With the kids, caretaking became a real issue. I had to take over a lot of that on short notice. Would I have to take the kids to school, fix lunch, fix dinner?

For the first couple of years, all sorts of crazy things went on around me. I was coping day-by-day, just getting by. I wasn't taking care of myself. I stuffed my feelings right and left. I had lots of experience doing that. I spent a lot of time numb, trying to keep everything under control. I tried to keep the household and the family stable, knowing that Sarah couldn't be counted on. I'm not putting her down for that. It was just a fact of life.

Sarah expressed thoughts of suicide every day for two years. It was scary. I had a lot of denial, "It won't really happen." But then I'd think, "What if it does? What can I do about it?" There would be times I'd wake up in the middle of the night and she would be gone and the car would be gone and I wouldn't know where she was. I'd have to have faith that she was safe. With two kids in the house, I couldn't go looking for her. She'd come home and say she'd been over on the coast on a cliff thinking about jumping off. I wouldn't know how to respond to that. I'd blank out. I'd tell her, "I'm happy you didn't jump." Inside, I'd be terrified. I was scared shitless each time she disappeared. It got to the point where I'd want a hug and kiss before she went anywhere. She'd be going to the store for a quart of milk and I'd kiddingly say, "I want a hug and kiss before you leave. I don't know if I'm going to see you again," but inside I'd be serious.

I was committed to Sarah. I was married to her. But there were times I asked myself, "What's going on? Is this worth it? Is this what a relationship is supposed to be—this constant chaos?" I wondered why I was staying in the relationship. What was in it for me? There was nothing in it for me at times. I entertained thoughts of quitting, but my commitment kept me there. I loved Sarah and we were going to get through this, but I kept watching things get worse and worse.

I started seeing her therapist, partly for my own issues, and more to keep track of where Sarah was at. To me, it seemed to me that she was getting way past the bounds of survivor healing. And I was going along blindly trusting this guy when this was happening. He kept assuring me, "Everything's fine. This is all normal. Everything will be fine in a year or two. . . ." It was kind of a carrot to keep me going.

"Things will be better." I guess I believed that. I trusted the guy. It turned out he was being sexually and emotionally inappropriate.

THERAPIST ABUSE

Sarah was in therapy with this man for a year and a half. He abused her during the last six months.

Most of Sarah's memories of the abuse were body memories. The way she expressed them to her therapist was to act them out through physical positions and motions. He started asking her to act out parts of the memories with him. He encouraged her to hit him, to lay on top of him, to express her desires for him. He actually said to Sarah at one point, "This is okay what we're doing, but of course, we can't do it out in the hall."

I didn't know the details of what he was doing, but I felt something was wrong. I asked him what was going on. He told me, "It's just transference. Once she's able to have these feelings for me, she'll be able to have them with you." I didn't know what he was talking about. When I found out what really happened, I was furious. I felt duped by the son of a bitch.

For Sarah, his abuse brought up the shame she'd felt as a child; but now she was feeling it as an adult. As her therapy with him continued, she became more and more suicidal. Eventually she began to wonder if what he was doing was right. She finally asked some other therapists, who told her therapy shouldn't be done that way; that she was being molested.

Sarah quit therapy with him and started working with a woman counselor. At first, Sarah doubted he'd really abused her, but eventually she got angry and worked up the courage to file a complaint with the state licensing board. They declined to file legal charges, saying there wasn't enough evidence. She also filed a complaint with the ethics committee of the statewide professional organization for therapists. They conducted an investigation; they interviewed the therapist and then they interviewed us. They wrote to us and told us they decided to discipline him, but they wouldn't tell us the nature of the discipline. We still don't know if they merely slapped his wrist, or if they fined him or pulled his license.

MEETING OTHER PARTNERS

From the very beginning, I needed support. I was confused and lonely. I assumed no one else in the world had these problems. It took two years for me to realize there were other survivors and other partners. I did the math one day: I figured one in three or four women are molested as children. That means there's a whole hell of a lot of partners out there, whether they know it or not. Half the men out here must be partners or have been partners of survivors and no one talks about it.

I saw a partners' workshop advertised and I went to it. Meeting other partners was a major turning point for me. I got a lot out of it. The fact that they felt the same way I did gave me a lot of validation and support.

I started a support group. It was great. I wished I'd had that from day one, from the first day that Sarah knew she'd been molested. A bunch of us got together. Some nights it would just be bitching and moaning about how bad things had been the past week with your survivor, how screwed up and crazy things were. We needed to get our feelings out. With the survivor, you can express some of that, but you have to be careful. With three or four other partners, you can let loose and all get pissed off together: "We haven't had sex in three months. This is nuts. I'm pissed off about it. This isn't what I got married for." After I got it out in the group, it was easier for me to get in touch with a gentler way of saying the same thing to Sarah.

Getting together with the group helped me form an identity as a partner. I got a lot of self-worth out of that identity. Lately, I haven't felt as much of a need to identify as a partner. Recently, I've been going to a men's support group. Most of them don't even know I'm a partner. As things have resolved, that label doesn't seem as important.

REVENGE FANTASIES

It took a while after Sarah remembered before she stopped seeing her father. She finally realized she couldn't maintain contact with him because he was denying everything and accusing her of being crazy. There was a lot of hassle with the family. It took two confrontations before Sarah was strong enough to stand up and say, "No, I'm not seeing you again."

It was hard for me to get angry at Sarah's father. I have a lot of parental respect; whatever parents say, goes. Parents are in a different category than other human beings. Getting angry at a parent is foreign to me. It took a while for me to get in touch with my anger at her father. I remember the time I did. I was in a partner's workshop, hearing the anger from all the other partners. I started getting into my own feelings. For the first time, I got angry at her father for what he'd done to Sarah and what he'd done to our relationship. It seems really ridiculous to want to punch out an old man, but I sure wanted to.

At one point, Sarah wanted to get some anger and hostility out. Being a contractor and a carpenter, I had hammers and blocks of wood and nails available. We drew a stick figure of her dad on a big chunk of wood and let her pound nails into it. I'd start the nails and then just let her swing as hard as she could to drive them in. She was so enthusiastic about pounding the nails in, I almost got my fingers crushed. Eventually she forgot the nails and just started bashing the piece of wood, just blew it apart. She obliterated the figure on the block of wood, just really got into it. She enjoyed it a lot.

I've got my own revenge fantasy going. I have a dress shirt her father gave me a couple of years ago. He always makes sure you know the value of his presents: he left the price tag on. It's a hundred-dollar dress shirt. I've never worn it. It's going to do me a lot of good to take it out and destroy it. I've thought of burning it, but that seems too quick. I want to destroy it slowly; to do something degrading to it at the same time. Shredding, maybe. Or dragging it around with the car, dreaming of him being in the shirt.

SEXUALITY

Our sexual relationship changed dramatically once the incest came out. Things got weird. It was difficult to initiate sex. Sarah would space out and go away. Other times she'd have to stop because she was having flashbacks.

After we had sex, she'd have this flood of emotion. It was disturbing for me. It seemed like I was doing something to Sarah to make her feel terrible. She wasn't supposed to feel terrible. She'd go to the bathroom after we had sex and throw up. How can you help but take that personally? I felt like a rapist sometimes, just having sex with my wife. I'd end up feeling terrible about the whole thing. It put a real damper on our sexual activity.

In a normal relationship, sexuality is a shared type of thing. But Sarah needed to control everything. Eventually we stopped having sex. There was so much hassle involved, I gave up. It just wasn't worth it.

I masturbated a lot. It was a fact of life. That was hard at first. Sarah and I were in a relationship together. We were supposed to do it together, not separately in different rooms at different times.

I bitched and moaned about it a lot. That's where the partners' group came in. We were all in the same boat.

I felt frustrated and angry. It helped to tell Sarah what I was feeling. She might not do anything differently, but the fact that she knew took some of the pressure off. But it was still hard for me to be patient. I kept pushing: "Let's fix it. Let's do something. Let's get this resolved."

Finally, we decided to establish a sexual moratorium where there'd be no sexual expectations whatsoever. If we wanted to talk about it, fine, but there wasn't going to be any pressure to do anything. We did that for four months. It was something we hadn't tried, and I was willing to try anything. Since we weren't having sex anyway, what difference did it make? I thought it might help. It did. It took the pressure off both of us. It allowed us to be safe with affection without expecting sexuality.

I tend to mix up affection and sexuality. With sex being so loaded, affection got screwed up too. There wasn't any physical affection, touching, or kidding around between us either. Everything became somber. Taking a break from sex gave us both an opportunity to feel safe with affection, knowing it wasn't going to lead to sex.

Sex is still the most difficult issue to deal with, the one we've put off till last to resolve. After we got through the first couple of years of crisis, we started working on sex, but we always had to stop. Sarah wouldn't feel safe enough. We'd put it off again. Every time we got close to dealing with this issue, bingo, another crisis came up to divert the focus. This has happened for the last two years. It's very frustrating to me.

Sarah has told me she wishes she never had to deal with sex

again; that if she was single she wouldn't have sex. Other times, she says she wants to work on it. Just recently, five years into her healing, she's been able to keep her focus on sexual issues. She's been able to stick with it.

We've been able to make progress in all kinds of other areas. We'll do it with sex too. It's just a matter of time.

I DIDN'T KNOW WHAT AN "ISSUE" WAS

Being the partner of a survivor has forced me to look at myself. Sarah was definitely learning about herself. The relationship wouldn't have worked if I hadn't done the same. I was forced to grow. I learned to look at my own issues and I didn't even know what an "issue" was. The first, most obvious one I had to look at was, "I don't have feelings." It's grown a lot from there.

I started out very dependent and eager to please Sarah. I always deferred to her. My stance was, "What can I do to help? What can I do for you?" Because of the lack of strong male figures in my childhood, I didn't have the confidence or strength to be myself, to put up something solid for Sarah to bump up against. Unless I assert myself, she has no idea who I am; it becomes easy for her to confuse me with her perpetrator. When I know who I am and what my limits are, I show her that I'm different: that I'm Eric and not her father. I give her something to lean on. It's been hard, but I'm learning to do that.

I've had to develop more assertiveness, the male masculinity side of me. I started standing up for myself more, asking for my needs to be met. I've learned to set limits. I'm starting to say no when I don't want to do something. Sarah says it feels better for her to know exactly where I stand. She feels safer. It's had a positive effect on her to realize, "You're here, too."

I think there's a dynamic at work that makes certain people connect with certain other people. Sarah didn't even know she was a survivor when we met and got married. The incest didn't come up until she was in a safe enough place to deal with it. She waited until our marriage. I took up the slack that allowed her the safety to go through this. It seems like more than a coincidence that I have issues in my background that affect her, too. We're discovering there's often a dynamic between the two.

HOW THINGS HAVE CHANGED

In the beginning, Sarah was in crisis constantly. We kept looking for things that would give us proof that things were improving. However small those things were, we focused on them.

After a couple of years, things started to stabilize. We started seeing more concrete progress. We could look back and say, "Look how much we've grown. Look how much we've accomplished. Look what we started with. Look where we are now. Who says there hasn't been any change?"

It hasn't been an easy five years, and I don't know if I'd do it again by choice. It's been difficult, but the adversity we've faced has built a lot of strength between us that might not have developed otherwise. Of course, I can't imagine doing it for anyone else but Sarah. That's what's made it so good: doing it with Sarah. I always felt that she was worth it. We have a good relationship now. It's getting stronger all the time.

LORRAINE'S STORY:
Breaking UP

Lorraine Williams was sexually abused by her grandfather. She was interviewed in 1984 for The Courage to Heal *about her experience confronting her family. The following interview picks up her story six years later, shortly after she ended a relationship with another survivor, Luci.*

When Luci and I met, I had come to a pretty solid place where I wasn't really dealing with the incest anymore. I had just left therapy after five years. I was feeling really good about myself. Being a survivor was no longer all-encompassing. The incest wasn't so much a part of my life. I had worked really hard, and through that work, I'd become capable of greater intimacy and fuller relationships.

I felt comfortable for the first time in my life with my sexuality, with being able to express it fully. I'd gotten to a place where I could really enjoy different facets of sex without feeling self-conscious or inhibited. I was trying new things. I no longer felt like I was a bad person or a terrible person because I liked sex. And I really like sex a lot.

When I met Luci, she was just beginning to look at the fact that she was having incest memories. She looked at it briefly, and then pushed it down again. She wasn't ready to deal with it. It wasn't until a year into the relationship that she really began to look at the incest and all her survivor issues came up.

Here was this person I loved and cared about who was having a hard time and lots of flashbacks. My first response was, "Okay, you're a survivor. We can deal with this." And I found myself asking questions like, "How does this affect you? How does this affect your sexuality?" I was distancing myself and being the therapist. Inside, I was going, "Oh, shit. I don't want to do this." But at the same time, I loved her. I was torn. I had a lot of unrealistic hopes: "I hope it wasn't as bad as my incest experience." "Well, maybe it won't take over her life." "Maybe she'll still want to be touched."

That's not what happened.

I wanted to be with somebody who was ready to be in a relationship, and all of a sudden, everything stopped. We fought. Sex stopped. Or we'd be making love and she'd fall into a flashback. I'd be lying there consoling her, and inside, I'd be fuming. I'd be on the verge of receiving this great pleasure and these damn incest memories would come up. It was frustrating. And it was a conflict because I felt I wasn't supposed to be angry. At times she said to me, "You're supposed to be understanding. You went through this." She expected me to have all the answers and I didn't.

The other thing that kept happening was that we'd make plans together, and she'd cancel. She wasn't able to be responsible or emotionally present. I was giving and giving and giving and not getting much back. She was capable of giving maybe ten percent.

I felt like I was with a walking zombie. It made me wonder, "Was I like that?" And I thought, "Nah, I couldn't have been like that," but I wasn't trying to be in a relationship while I went through it.

I was angry. I'd spent all this time working on me, and now I get involved with someone who's broken? Now I'm supposed to start back at the beginning again?

I grew increasingly impatient. I felt I owed it to the relationship to be patient and to offer her my support. In actuality, I didn't want anything to do with it. I was tired of incest. I didn't want to be in a relationship with someone who was broken. I didn't want to have to wait all that time for her to go through the healing process, through all the "Don't touch me's. I can't handle this," the outbursts of crying, the "I'm shut down," all of it. I didn't want to go through years of that. And I knew that when she was done, she might not want to have anything to do with me. It was too big a risk.

I tried to wait and hold out, to be there and hold her. I'd think,

"This is what a partner is supposed to do." I tried to make it okay that I wasn't getting a lot of gratification, but I wasn't getting my needs met at all. I felt terribly isolated.

I felt a tremendous amount of guilt. I thought, "I should be more understanding. I've been through this." I thought about how wonderful it would have been to have someone who'd been understanding for me. Then I'd feel like a terrible person. I'd ask myself, "How come I can't give this to her? Why can't I do this." And another part of me would answer, "I can't do this. I don't want to do this." It was just too draining. I'd ask myself, "Am I being selfish?" And I'd answer, "Yes, I am being selfish." Sometimes that felt okay and sometimes it didn't.

Things finally came to a head over the holidays. They were horrible. We were supposed to spend Christmas Eve together. She went to do a gift exchange with some other friends. I stayed at her house and did laundry. We were preparing to go out of town the next day. I was sitting and listening to music, and it came to me: "She's not coming home." She called a half hour later to say she wasn't coming home because she didn't feel emotionally strong enough to face the world and travel. She said if she tried she would either get drunk or commit suicide.

I wasn't surprised. I was hurt and angry and disappointed, but I wasn't surprised. That night, I came to the conclusion it wasn't worth it for me to stay in the relationship. It wasn't worth it being disappointed all the time. I'd put a lot of energy out, more than one hundred percent, and what I received in return was pain and anguish and torment. I didn't want to be a martyr.

When she came home the next morning, she hugged me and kissed me and said, "I know you're angry." I had decided to put the anger on hold so we could spend Christmas Day together. I managed to put it on hold for a few hours. Then we had to talk. I said, "It just hurts too much."

We did go away together. It was an okay vacation, but there was no physical intimacy. There was no lovemaking. That had stopped at Thanksgiving. I was feeling very, very deprived.

When we came back from that vacation, we'd both done a lot of thinking. We both realized being together wasn't possible. It finally sunk into my brain that Luci wasn't available, and that she probably wasn't going to be available for a long time. I'd been telling myself it would get better, that we'd get through it, that it would soon be over. What I recognized then was that we weren't even close to it being over. I realized I didn't have what it took to stick it out. That didn't mean I didn't love her or want to be with her. It just meant that it was too painful for me, and ultimately too painful for her, because she didn't have anything to give. She felt like a failure because she kept disappointing and hurting me. She didn't want to continue to hurt me. And I knew if I stayed I would end up resenting her. And I didn't want to do that. I didn't want to end up hating her.

I wanted it to be over.

It hurt, but it was a good ending. We both knew it wasn't working and there was nothing we could do about it. We spent a long time holding one another and crying. We knew this was what we had to do.

I spent more time crying within the relationship than I did when it actually ended. I did so much grieving for things that had been lost while we were together that I didn't have many tears left when we finally broke up.

For the next month or so, I backed off from her. We didn't see each other much at all, maybe twice in a month. I had a lot of anger, lots of revenge fantasies toward her. I felt like I'd been robbed, that she'd just taken from me and not given anything back.

Luci was in therapy dealing with incest, and started to look at her part in the relationship ending. Eventually she was able to acknowledge she'd hurt me a lot. From that point on, we were able to work at having a friendship. The quality of our friendship is better now than it was when we were lovers. She's more capable of following through because she's further along in her healing process. I have fewer expectations of her. There's less pressure on her to be intimate.

I'm sure I said to friends, "I'm not getting involved with any more incest survivors at the beginning of their work." That's a difficult decision to make since so many lesbians are incest survivors, but I've been successful. I'm involved with someone now who's not an incest survivor. It's nice to know we're going to be able to make love without this third person who caused damage coming in to interrupt things. I'm much happier now. I'm sure I made the right decision.

RICHARD'S STORY:
A Year at a Time

Richard and Yvonne are in their midthirties. Richard is a CPA and Yvonne is a criminal attorney. They've been married twelve years and have no children. Yvonne was sexually and ritually abused in a cult that included her parents.

I grew up in the Midwest, the youngest of three children. My mother was somewhat domineering and my father let her have her way. Emotions were looked down on in my family. No one showed affection. My mother-in-law was the first person who ever hugged and kissed me as an adult.

I met Yvonne during our freshman year in college. The first thing that attracted me to Yvonne was her intelligence. She's a brilliant woman; that really excited me. I was feeling lonely and isolated; I'd never gone out on a date before. I had very little experience with women and, as a result, made all kinds of mistakes when we were first together. After we'd been dating for about a year, I put a lot of pressure on Yvonne to have sex with me. She eventually gave in. It was a bad experience for both of us. She was scared and I felt guilty afterwards.

It was hard, but it didn't break us up. We continued to have sex, and eventually got married. We agreed not to have kids; we wanted to focus on our careers. We put Yvonne's career on the front burner; it took precedence and it continues to do so. I'm glad we did it that way.

Five years into our marriage, Yvonne started having night-mares. Sex started to go badly. I couldn't please her; her sexual interest in me was waning. I thought there was something wrong with me. I felt very mixed up. I'd never had sex with anyone else. I kept thinking, "Is this what sex is supposed to be like? Is this all I can look forward to for the rest of my life?"

I got this idea that if Yvonne had sex with someone else, it might help. We got involved with a friend of mine in a three-way relationship. After six months, he moved in with us. The whole thing lasted a year. We finally kicked him out, but by that time, Yvonne was so confused she moved out, too. It was a colossal mess, and it almost broke up our marriage.

I got into therapy. I asked Yvonne to join me, and told her I didn't hold much hope for our marriage if she didn't. We started going to couples' counseling. My goal was to get back together. Hers was to sort things out and see what she really wanted. We worked on issues of communication, boundaries, and setting limits. Most of it was new for us.

After four or five months, we moved back in together. We kept going to counseling, both individually and together. It was during one of her sessions alone with our therapist that Yvonne began to remember and reveal the sexual abuse. She told me about it in a very gradual way. It was like peeling an onion. It still is.

At first, I tried to be really supportive. I wanted to take the burden from her; to share the pain. I was in there fighting with her every step of the way.

I attended several workshops for partners of survivors. Every-one was in a lot of pain, and until then, I hadn't realized how much pain I was in. Everyone in the group was trying to be superhuman; none of us were happy. There was an incredible rate of burnout. At one point, there were eight of us meeting once a week, and after six months, all but two of the couples had split up. That had quite an impact on me. I said to myself, "These guys are really letting them-selves get screwed over and pushed around." The men were all very giving, too giving. Where did it get them? They ended up with bro-ken relationships.

I realized I was trying to be there too much for Yvonne. I couldn't keep trying to feel her feelings while my own needs for intimacy and sexuality went unmet. I stopped trying to share in her pain. By this time, Yvonne had developed a wide network of women friends, She'd worked with several therapists. I started letting her rely on her own support network more. Our relationship is healthier now because of that.

HAVING AFFAIRS

It seems to me that the more Yvonne reveals and remembers, the worse our sex life gets. Yvonne can have sex with me, but she's never been able to kiss me deeply and intimately. Having people or objects close to her face really freaks her out. I've had a hard time coming to grips with that. It still feels like rejection.

Several years after the abuse surfaced, I had an affair with a mutual friend. I wasn't out to hurt Yvonne or to make a statement. I had just turned thirty and Yvonne was the only woman I'd ever been with. I wanted to know if sex would feel different with someone else.

It was a one-time affair, yet it created a new frame of reference for me. I'd never realized someone could desire me that way. I suddenly felt adequate and I'd never felt that with Yvonne. I realized sex could be very different than what I was experiencing in my marriage.

I must have been hell to live with. I fell in love with this other woman. I was so excited I couldn't work for several days. It felt like something wonderful had been revealed to me.

I told Yvonne about the affair right away. In fact, I kept telling her what a great experience it had been. I was very naive. I thought she'd be happy for me. Instead, she was jealous and hurt. The more I described the wonderful sex we'd had, the more inadequate Yvonne felt. Mostly, I think, she was afraid of being compared to this other woman.

In some ways, though, the affair made things easier between us. I was able to ease up on my expectations of Yvonne. I wasn't as demanding as I might have been otherwise. I felt like I had been filled. Even though intimacy and sex weren't that great with Yvonne for the next few years, the good feelings from the affair carried me for a long time.

But eventually, our communication around sex broke down.

Initially we'd given a lot of airtime to sex in our therapist's office, but later Yvonne kept wanting to work on other issues instead. I felt totally misunderstood; that Yvonne had no understanding of what I needed.

Less than a year ago, I had a second affair. The woman was a friend; we spent one night together in a hotel. I didn't enter into it lightly. I knew what was at stake and it wasn't easy. I felt guilty, ashamed, and scared. I knew I was going to tell Yvonne about it and I wasn't sure what her reaction would be. I knew she might kick me out of the house, but I still needed to do it. It sounds horrible, but the fix I'd acquired from the first affair was wearing off. I'd forgotten what it was like to have someone really desire me.

I came back from the weekend and told Yvonne immediately. At first, she was dumbfounded. She couldn't believe it. Then she got really angry. She said she didn't want to be in the relationship anymore.

After the real heavy anger, Yvonne did a lot of things right. She set limits. She said I couldn't talk to the woman while we were working things out. She insisted that we get back into couples' counseling (we had stopped for a while), and that we focus more on issues from my past. She said she didn't want me having any more affairs.

After the smoke cleared, we did talk more honestly about sex. Yvonne didn't condone what I did, but she was able to acknowledge that she really hadn't acknowledged the depth of my sexual frustration. A couple of years ago she used to tell me I was oversexed and abnormal because I wanted sex more than once a week. That drove me crazy. Now, she's willing to say that my sexual needs are legitimate.

Right now Yvonne's dealing with some really heavy memories, and she's made it clear I shouldn't expect a lot of change around sex in the near future. She's not ready to deal with sexual issues; she's already got a full agenda to work with. I'm glad she can finally tell me where she is, but I'm still not getting what I need. For now, I can live with that. I'm a lot more patient than I used to be.

FUTURE THOUGHTS

I used to think about the future a lot; where I would be in ten years, whether this relationship was right for me. Now I only think of things a few months or a year at a time. That's upsetting for Yvonne. She wants more of a commitment than that. But that's my limit. I can't give her an unqualified commitment. I can't say, "Yes, I'll always be here for you."

For many years, I didn't consider leaving my marriage a possibility. I didn't feel I had a choice. It got so bad that I started having fantasies of Yvonne dying in a car accident. I didn't want her to die, but it was the only way I could imagine getting out of the relationship—either she'd leave me or there'd be an accident. When I caught myself having weird thoughts about her dying, I realized I had to give myself the option to leave. I had to tell myself I wasn't a bad person for thinking about it. And I wouldn't be a bad person if I did decide to leave.

I've tested the waters. I've talked to friends who've been through divorce. Yvonne and I talk about it from time to time. We've both questioned whether being together is the best thing for us. But we're very good friends. We have a lot of history. I love being with someone as intelligent and caring and compassionate as Yvonne. That's a big incentive to stay together. I want more, but for now it's enough to carry me.

WHY IT'S BEEN WORTH IT

I may decide to call it quits one day, but I'll never regret having been in this relationship. It's been difficult, but I've grown tremendously; I wouldn't be the same person if I hadn't spent the last twelve years with Yvonne. I'd be a lot less mature. That maturity has been painful, but it's been worth it.

Sometimes I gloss over the progress we've made over the years, the difficult issues we've weathered, but really we both deserve a pat on the back. I'm proud of the things we've done. Most couples would have called it quits after the affairs; we were able to work it through.

Our emotional growth has been a leapfrogging process for us; sometimes I'm able to see things more clearly, and my clarity helps move us ahead; other times Yvonne is the one who's leading the way. When we get bogged down on difficult issues, she's the one who usually cuts through the muck and gets us back on track. I'm very proud of her for that.

I love Yvonne. She's gone through hell and I have tremendous respect for the process she's going through. I love the connection Yvonne has with life—with people and with animals. She inspires me. She's like a flower in the process of blossoming.

SCOTT'S STORY:
Building Trust
over Time

*Scott and his partner, Jim, have been lovers for eight years. They live in the
Boston area and are about to live together for the first time. Scott, thirty-six,
ran his own cleaning business for years and is currently on disability. Jim,
thirty-two, is a counselor. Jim was sexually abused by his father.*

I grew up in the Midwest. My father was an evangelical Baptist
minister. He was an interim pastor, so we moved a great deal. We
lived in South Dakota and Oklahoma and Kansas and everywhere
in between.

My mother hated being a preacher's wife. She took her frustration out on us. She abused me and my sister in every possible way,
except sexually. One time, she beat me so badly I had to go to the
hospital. She chased me with a butcher knife, but of course, who
would have believed a preacher's wife could do such things?

I've spent most of my life in therapy trying to figure out why
my mother abused me. I felt terribly cheated. I kept asking, "Why?
Why didn't I have Jane Wyatt as a mother? Why didn't I grow up
on 'Father Knows Best'?" I had a lot of anger about it. I've gotten to
a point now where I've confronted her. We are in the long process
of evaluating what the abuse meant to us. She's in therapy now, too,
and she's acknowledged a lot of her own problems.

My father was basically a passive man. He never did anything
to stop my mother's abuse. Before he died a year ago, I talked to

him about what she did to me. For the first time, he was able to validate a lot of it. He held me and told me he loved me. I feel at peace with him now.

THE EARLY YEARS

I married a woman right out of high school. But I kept having these feelings for men. I thought I was the only gay man in the whole world. It wasn't something anyone talked about, particularly not in the Bible Belt. Finally, I went to my wife and told her. I said, "I'm different and I can't handle a marriage." I think I expected her to save me and she expected me to acquiesce to the marriage. It just didn't work. There was a lot of anger on both our parts. Finally, after three years, we dissolved the marriage.

It was very hard for my mother to deal with the fact that I was gay. She treated it like a disease and felt she was somehow responsible. She forbade me to come into her home. It was probably the best thing she ever did for me because I finally got some distance from her.

From the time I came out, at twenty-two, I lived a fairly stereotypically gay lifestyle. I've always been relationship-oriented. I've always been looking for love. I went from relationship to relationship, never really getting too far because I kept choosing people who would abuse me. I put myself in abusive situations because it's all I'd ever known.

When I met Jim, I was just starting to deal with the fact that I'd been abused by my mother. He was ready to face the incest with his father. For the first month we were together, our connection was around our abuse. We were both having memories. We cried a lot together. We hurt a lot together. It was very cathartic. The relationship was a place where we could both unload. During the first six months of our relationship, a lot came out.

It made our relationship feel crazy. I got a lot of mixed messages from Jim. I'd see him one time and he'd be very warm and open to me, and the next time, he'd be really hostile and angry. He'd say, "I love you. Come near me." Then when I'd come near him, he'd push me away with a great deal of force. He was terribly confused. What he felt was, "I love you and I want to trust you, but you're going to hurt me like my father did."

At the beginning of our relationship, I was a clothing model in New York. I was making a lot of money. Unbeknownst to him, I made all these arrangements for us to be together: fancy hotel suites and roses and champagne and limousines and tickets to see *Cats,* which was playing on Broadway. He felt threatened and overwhelmed by all the attention. He called my roommate and left a message, "Tell Scott I can't do it." And then he ran away. I spent a miserable weekend alone in New York.

I loved him and wanted to be close to him. And I pushed for that. And the more I pushed, the more he ran away.

Jim kept mistaking my affection for an act of perpetration. He had very strong reactions to my attention to him, particularly in a physical way. He had a lot of trouble separating me from his father. I was constantly being told I was the perpetrator.

One time, early in our relationship, I went to see him on New Year's Eve. He was having some friends over. I went over and gave him a great big kiss. He looked at me and he said, "How dare you do that! How dare you treat me that way!" And I said, "What way?" To me, it felt natural and normal. I was just being affectionate. As far as he was concerned, it was an act of perpetration. I felt confused and angry. I stood up to him and said, "That's not me. You should be getting angry at the person who hurt you, not at me."

After each of these incidents, we'd both be angry and we'd retreat to our separate corners to lick our wounds. Sometimes that would be for a few days. Sometimes it would be as long as six months. And that happened for the first four or five years of our relationship.

When we took time apart, it would help me get clearer about who I was as a person. I'd sit down with myself and say, "Hey, I'm not a perpetrator. I feel affection for Jim. I'm not trying to control him. I love him and care about him. This is a growing relationship." And Jim would get a chance to take a look at who he was and who I was in his life.

We both initiated these times apart. I could see them coming. He would be very threatened by my sexuality. He'd get more and more uncomfortable being near me. It would keep escalating. There was nothing I could do. He would finally tell me to get away.

He'd reject me and tell me I wasn't worth it. These were things I'd heard all my life.

One time we'd been bickering and fighting for quite a while. I was very confused and hurt by it, and finally I called him and said, "Jim, I need to come over and talk to you." I went over and said, "I need some space from you. I really care about you, but I'm feeling bad about myself. I need some time to sort through the things you've been saying to me." He got angry and felt I was abandoning him. There was a lot of hurt involved.

During our separations, we sometimes corresponded through letters. Phone calls didn't work. Sometimes it was too risky for him even just to hear my voice. He hung up on me all the time. He was in love with me and he was afraid that our love would control him. Telling him I was different than his father wasn't enough. He had to see it.

During our separations, going out with other men was a given for me. I tried to substitute other people for Jim. But each time I did, I realized it wasn't really what I wanted. I was in love with him. I wanted him.

Having other relationships wasn't a priority for Jim. He dated other men sometimes, but other times he'd be celibate. It felt good for him not to feel forced to perform sexually.

Each time we got back together, we'd have to get through the things that had happened while we were apart. He'd feel jealous of the men I'd been with. I had my share of those feelings, too.

In the beginning, it seemed like we were breaking up each time we took time apart. We didn't know how to say, "We need a break from each other." Later in our relationship, as we got closer and more trust was built, we were able to say, "We both need some space from each other," and there wouldn't be so much hurt attached.

TWO HURT LITTLE BOYS

I think sometimes sexually abused people feel entitled: "I was hurt so I'm entitled to act this way." He felt he had carte blanche to be a naughty boy all the time. And that wasn't okay with me. I told him, "I'm really sorry about what happened to you. But just because you were abused doesn't give you the right to abuse me." And he'd say, "You're absolutely right, but I still want to do it." And I'd say, "That's too bad. I have rights, too." Then we'd laugh.

Humor has been important to us. The ability to look at yourself and laugh; to be able to say, "Did I *really* say that?" This is a very serious subject, but there have been times it's been really funny.

He has a hurt little boy inside of him, and I have a hurt little boy inside of me. Sometimes he'll say to me, "I *hate* you." And I'll say, "I *hate* you, too!" And then we'll both laugh. It's clearly not the adults who love each other talking here. It's the two hurt little boys.

We've found that both of us being abused could either be a very big plus or a very big minus. We understood each other's pain. We could comfort each other. But we also knew how to hurt each other. There were times when we were destroying each other, when we weren't building anything between us. We'd get into these giant fights over control. Neither of us ever had any control in our lives, so naturally we both wanted as much as we could get.

We had a terrible shouting match one time. He was screaming, "I was terribly abused. I'm a victim and that's all there is to it. You're going to have to do exactly what I want or I can't go on with this relationship!" And I said, "But *I've* been abused and I'm a victim, too, and you're going to have to go along with me." He said, "Well, I can't do that." And I said, "Well, I can't either." We were at a standstill and separated for a period of time.

Then he came back to me and he said, "You know what? We're both acting like victims, aren't we?" And I said, "Yeah. And you know what? We're not victims. We're survivors. And that's the difference." We were able to turn that experience around and learn from it. But it wasn't easy. We both had to let go of a lot of pain and take a risk. We had to give up the label of victim. And we had to trust each other. Given our backgrounds, that was very difficult.

Even though there were times he said, "I don't love you," I always knew we loved each other. I remember one time in particular. We were sitting in the car. We hadn't seen each other in a while. And he said to me, "I'm not sure I want a primary relationship in my life right now." He was very arrogant about it. And I looked at him and I said, "Oh really? I think you better take another look. I think you already have one." The question I was putting to him was, "Are you ready to accept the fact that this is true?" I knew it was true, and on some level, he knew it was, too. But he fought it.

He used to say, "If I give in to you, you will have won." And I used to say, "Won? What am I winning? Am I winning an award? Am I winning the lottery? What did I win?" He'd say, "You'll have succeeded in breaking me down." I'd say, "That's not what I want at all. I want you to be the happiest you can be, whether you're with me or not."

That day in the car, after I asked him point-blank, he looked at me, and we both laughed. Finally, there was a degree of acceptance.

MEN ARE SUPPOSED TO BE SEXUAL

Men expect other men to be sexual. It's the way we've been socialized. It's one of the big conflicts Jim has had with me. I'm a very sexual man. I have been all my life. I'm a good-looking gay man, and I've always gotten a lot of acceptance at that level. Because of the dysfunction in my family, I was always looking for love. So I was having sex all the time.

With Jim, being sexual is a love-hate thing. He's attracted to men and it was a man who abused him. That's hard for him. He's given me so many mixed messages about sex because there's a healthy side of him and an unhealthy side that have been constantly warring. Sometimes he accepts me. He'd say, "You're a virile gay man, Scott, and I really love that." And then ten minutes later, he'd say, "I hate you because you're a virile man." It's been terribly confusing for both of us. I never knew where he was going to be or how long he'd be there.

We'd be making love, and everything would be fine, and then out of nowhere, he would freeze up and everything would stop. At first I got really frustrated and angry. Then we started talking our way through it. That involved a lot of risk for both of us. He'd say, "I'm feeling very frightened. I don't know where it's coming from." Just saying that would help him relax. I'd say to him, "This doesn't feel so great for me either. I don't want you to feel forced to do anything. I want this to be how we naturally feel about each other. I'd rather we don't go on at all than go on with forced sex."

Understandably, he needed a lot of control around sex. We had sex when he felt like it. It felt to me like I had to be at his beck and call. I resented that deeply. I finally was able to make him understand that I didn't want to be used any more than he did.

AIDS AND INCEST

I was diagnosed with AIDS a year ago. I was in the hospital with pneumocystis pneumonia. I'd been diagnosed with ARC (AIDS-Related-Complex) for a year before that, but was only mildly symptomatic. Jim is HIV positive, but only has a few mild symptoms.

My AIDS diagnosis has changed things. This is a life-threatening disease and we've risen to the challenge in our lives. It's put incest on the back burner. It's still there, but it doesn't have the power it once did. Part of that is all the work we've done. Part of it is dealing with something so much more immediate.

There have been other changes as well. Jim was used to calling the shots around sex for such a long time. All of a sudden, it's out of his control. I'm the one saying no. There have been times I just haven't felt sexual. And Jim doesn't know what to do with that, because I'd always been available before. Saying no to him from my side of things has been good for both of us, I think. He's realized that he isn't in control. It's not so important anymore.

One of the things AIDS robs people of is your dignity. I haven't been able to work. I'm on disability now. We're trying to get subsidized housing right now. Dealing with Medicaid and Social Services has been really hard.

We're about to move in together. That's new. We used to say to each other, "I'll never live with you." Then it was, "When and if we ever live with each other." Then it went to, "When we live with each other." And now it's, "We are going to live with each other." That progression parallels our growth as a couple. It feels like things have finally reached fruition. We've reached a point in our lives where we can say, "We really deserve to be the couple that we have been working so hard to be for the last eight years." There's a lot of joy in that. But the shadow of AIDS is there. Jim has said to me, "I've been afraid to live with you because if I live with you, that would mean that you would die."

We've discussed this pretty thoroughly, and I think we both agree that this is a beginning. Whether I live or I die, or whether he lives or he dies, we will have had this. We'll have the satisfaction of knowing we reached this level of intimacy. We've both worked very hard at this. And we'll continue to grow together. That's the joy of it.

This has been a great life experience for me. It could have been a disaster if I hadn't been ready for it in my life. But I was solid enough in myself to sustain the constant barrage of testing. "Do you really love me or are you just using me?" That question got asked over and over again, in a million different ways. He threw the kitchen sink at me.

I've learned to trust. I've learned patience. I've also learned how to be there for someone without giving up on myself. I learned when to let go. I learned that when you let go of someone, that's when you're really ready to have them. When you're at the point when you can say, "It's really not all that important," you're really secure enough with yourself to receive.

I've learned negotiation, which is something I didn't know any-thing about. We deal with issues much faster now. It used to take us four months to do what we can now do in an hour. Five or six years ago, we would have to retreat to our corners. Now it's a lot easier, and we can work things out together. If we need space now, we can say that and spend time apart, but it's not a fracturing of the rela-tionship: "I have a relationship. I don't have a relationship. I have a relationship. I don't have a relationship." There's a lot more cohe-siveness to things now.

The defensiveness is gone. Now when an incest-related thing comes up, he's much more willing to say, "Oh God, this is an incest thing, isn't it?" And I'll say, "Sure smells like it to me."

A lot of things have come back around full circle. We went to see *Cats* last Wednesday in Boston. It wasn't the same, but we were finally able to see it together. I had carried a lot of animosity about that experience, and he felt a lot of guilt. We talked about it after the show and we were finally able to let it go. It was really nice. There have been a number of things like that, that we've had to go back and heal.

I'm very proud of us. I'm proud that I stuck it out. There were so many times it would have been easy to just turn and walk away.

SCOTT'S STORY: BUILDING TRUST OVER TIME

And I'm glad I didn't. My instincts were right. He was worth it. I'm glad I believed in the love we had between us. It was very real, and it continues to be. I love him as much, if not more, than I did eight years ago. I think that's pretty remarkable. For all its pain, it's been an incredible experience.

VIRGINIA'S STORY:
Forging a
Commitment

Virginia is fifty years old. Her husband, Keith, is fifty-three. They've been married for twenty years. They have six children, two from her first marriage, and four together. The three oldest have left home. Two teenage daughters and a nine-year-old son live with them in their sprawling Minneapolis home. Virginia worked with battered women for twelve years. Now she is a painter, and her husband Keith, an engineer. Keith was abused by both parents and his grandparents as well, and has been dealing with specific memories of sexual abuse for the last three years.

    I grew up in a working-class family on both sides: my mother left high school and worked in a factory when she was fifteen; my father also started work in a factory. I was part Indian on both sides. When I was growing up, my parents were in the process of disembodying their roots. They were trying to make it into the middle class and leave their history behind. The price they paid for that was a lot of alcohol abuse. My mother was an alcoholic. My brother became an instant alcoholic at sixteen. My father drank too much, and later developed a dependency on drugs. I was the only person not abusing alcohol in my family.

    My role was to take care of everybody. When my brother tried to kill himself at age sixteen, my mother told me it was because I'd gone away to college. I was devastated. I was the classic caretaker. I've done a lot of work around that. I've been in Al-Anon for many years.

By the time I met Keith, more than ten years later, I was a divorced mother with two kids. I was hiding out in St. Paul, living under a fake name, trying to escape from my first husband, who beat me. It was before anyone talked about battered women. I thought it was all my fault.

I was going to a drop-in therapy group and that's where I met Keith. We became friends at first. Six months after the group ended, we started seeing each other.

Before I met Keith, he'd been institutionalized several times with a diagnosis of schizophrenia. He told me about it soon after we met. Keith doesn't hide things. I was concerned about the hereditary aspect of schizophrenia and I read up on it. I asked people a lot of questions. About a third of schizophrenics spontaneously recover and he seemed to be one of those. He didn't need drugs. He seemed to be fine. But I was still worried, so we drove up to the hospital he'd been in and I talked to the doctor. I wanted to know how safe he was. She was reassuring. She said he was in good shape. She'd really worked wonders with Keith, helped make him into a terrific person. But of course she never asked about sexual abuse. Nobody talked about these things the way they do now. No one ever asked the right questions. It just wasn't in the culture.

THE EARLY YEARS

The main problem in my relationship with Keith was the fact that I wanted to control him. I'd been used to caretaking my parents and my brother. I wanted to take care of Keith and control him. And I would get angry when I couldn't do that.

I began moving out of that years ago when I started going to feminist consciousness-raising groups. I stopped being so interested in taking care of Keith and started demanding that he do his share around the house and with the kids. We had the usual battle about that. For the most part, he's been very receptive.

Twelve years ago, a friend of mine killed herself. My best friend said to me at the time, "What makes you think you had the power to save her life?" That was very potent for me. I started to peel off another whole level of caretaking behavior. I let Keith run his own life and make his own mistakes. I started to treat him like an adult, not like a child.

Keith has always had problems with work. Each time there'd be a specific problem, so we'd focus on that, instead of recognizing he had a pattern of difficulties. He's a brilliant man, very good at what he does, but he's always felt this nameless dread at work. He kept having these massive panic attacks around work. What would happen is that he would have trouble, and then I'd give him an ultimatum, and he'd pull it together.

Work seems to be the one area in which the abuse affects him. It's quite a miracle. He's never been abusive toward the kids. He's a wonderful lover. Sex with Keith has always been one of the best parts of our marriage. He wins all the feminist awards in that category. He's very tender. Nothing depends on his penis. He seems to set aside whatever anxiety he feels when we're in bed together. I read all the books, and I always feel, "He's better than anything in the books." Sex has been a great comfort to us. It's the glue that's helped us through recovery.

For a while after the abuse surfaced, neither of us could think of a single damned thing to say to each other. Every topic was taboo. I said, "Don't tell me any flashbacks." And he didn't want to hear me lecture him or tell him how to run his life. For a while, if I wasn't lecturing him, it was very tough to think of anything to say. We could barely talk about the weather. But we could stay in touch physically, and that's been a wonderful comfort to us.

THE MEMORIES STARTED COMING

The cataclysmic event that led to the sexual abuse coming out was my father's death. It really affected both of us. It threw me into therapy and it disoriented Keith. He started having another round of problems at work. On Sunday night or Monday morning, before he had to go to work, he'd start to panic. At work, he'd be overcome with tremendous waves of fear. He'd feel like someone was standing over his shoulder about to attack him. He was fearful of his boss, in a real state of terror. It was inexplicable. He hated going to work.

Finally, I encouraged him to quit, and he did. He was under extreme stress and started going to therapy.

We didn't understand what was going on until he'd been in therapy for a number of months. We thought he was seeking help for his work problems. But six months after he started, he began to have memories of sexual abuse.

Keith always knew he'd been treated horribly. He knew his parents didn't want him. As a child, he heard his mother say many times that she'd wanted to abort him. At fourteen, he overheard his parents saying they wanted to have a son, as if he didn't exist.

So Keith knew he was unwanted and hated, and he knew his father battered his mother horribly. When she was nine months pregnant with his brother, he remembers his father beating her bloody in the utility room and the ambulance coming. His father was violent toward all of them. And Keith's mother is a drug addict. She's been addicted to uppers and downers for at least thirty years. By the time he was in college, Keith figured out from her medications that she was probably schizophrenic as well.

He lived with his parents for his first five years. Then he moved in with his grandparents because his parents didn't want him anymore. Keith always thought of his grandparents as his saviors. They basically raised him. He was like a son to them. He blanked out the rest.

The first thing Keith remembered in therapy was that his mother tried to drown him as a baby. His grandmother came in and saved him. He also remembered his grandmother pulling down his pants when he was a little toddler, checking for bruises and blood. Then he remembered his father sexually abusing him, and later, his grandmother doing the same. If Keith had sex with his grandmother, she'd promise to keep his mother from killing him. This was before he was eight years old.

About the time he was having these memories, we went to see Keith's younger sister. She told us that Keith's father used to beat up their mother and then sexually abuse her. She told us about times she remembered Keith's father beating him. And she told us about the time she was twelve years old and told to potty train her much younger brother. Her mother pulled down the baby's pants and his penis was bloody and bruised. She turned to the sister and accused her of doing it. She said, "You're doing a horrible job. You're being rough when you're potty training him."

MULTIPLE PERSONALITIES

Last summer, Keith's therapist told him he had multiple personalities, but he didn't tell me until January. I freaked out. I have not seen any multiple personalities. They seem to be confined to his therapist's office. Sometimes when he's anxious in the morning, he'll call his therapist from the office, and she'll say, "Let me talk to the person who handles work." I haven't had the impulse to do that, because I don't see different people. I've thought a lot about it. I see him anxious at times. I see him depressed. I see him self-absorbed, but I don't see someone different coming out. Keith feels that he doesn't do it at home either, that it happens within the confines of therapy.

Keith and I have this agreement that our therapists can talk to each other. I had my therapist ask his therapist, "Are any of these personalities dangerous? Could he ever flip out and hurt me or the kids?" His therapist said, "Don't worry. He's safe. He's not dangerous in any way." That reassured me, but it's still hard for me to deal with.

Not much surprises me. I ran safe houses for battered women for twelve years and I had to report child abuse. But the news that he had multiple personalities was devastating to me. I thought, "I don't want to live with a crazy man. I've had it." Keith and I had a long talk about it. I went through being furious. I said, "Fuck this. This is the last straw." Then I went through feeling silly and giddy about it. "Oh great! How many of you are there and what are their names?" Finally I said, "Move out. Take you and you and all the rest of you out of here!" But we just kept talking and by the time we finished, I was able to say, "I don't care if there are a hundred of you. I want you to help out with the kids. I want you to cook dinner. I want you to think about me. I want all the same things I wanted before I found out about this, and if you can do those things, we can work it out."

Maybe someday this multiple personality thing is going to be of paramount importance, but right now, I'm concerned with the basic issues that exist between partners who are trying to share a life as two adults and share responsibility for children. I told him, "I don't even think I can keep my mind focused on what multiple personalities are, and in a way, I'm not interested. I'm interested in your behavior, the behavior between you and me." I live in the here and now, and the fact is, he's been doing pretty well. If he can keep it up, that's all I really care about.

AND THEY KEPT COMING

About a year and a half ago, Keith went back to work. It's still very hard for him. Most of his flashbacks have occurred at work. It's devastating for him. He has a professional position, and there he is at his desk, feeling like a terrified two-year-old.

Just this past spring, he had a horrible memory. When he was a baby and his parents and grandparents and he all lived together, his mother's cousin Jane, who was dying from meningitis, lived with them. He really loved this cousin; that much he always remembered. What came up for him was that she'd been lying on the sofa one day, in tremendous pain, begging someone to kill her. Keith was two years old. Jane told him to go in the kitchen and get a knife. He went into the kitchen and got a knife. The weapons were supposed to be out of her way, but this was clearly a setup by his family. He brought the knife to her, she put her hands around his hands, pushed the knife through her heart, and died.

When his mother and his grandmother came in, his mother picked him up and threw him against the wall, saying he was a murderer and that he should be killed. She asked, "How are we going to do it?" And his grandmother replied, "We're not going to kill him. We're just going to make him suffer. It's better to make him suffer." So after that, it didn't matter to any of them what they did to him. They considered him a murderer.

Keith remembered this whole scene absolutely clearly. It's amazing to me that he can remember every detail and he was only two years old. Really, it's amazing he survived at all.

Just recently, he's begun to remember ritual abuse. His grandfather was a fundamentalist, lots of fire and damnation. So far, Keith has only bits and pieces. He thinks he witnessed murders, and that his grandfather was responsible. But he doesn't have a clear memory like he does with his cousin. It's all still a tangle.

The ritual abuse memories have flipped him out. It's been difficult for him at work again. He started seeing his therapist twice a week, and they cut off dealing with the ritual abuse memories for now, so he can focus more on stabilizing his life at work.

So far, we haven't been able to figure out why these memories only come up at work. There must be some kind of trigger. The understanding we have so far, the one that makes sense to us, is that Keith doesn't want to hurt us at home. The most important thing to him is me and the kids. If the abuse has to come out, he'd rather be hurt at work.

TALKING TO THE KIDS

The whole time Keith wasn't working, he wouldn't tell the kids why. And the older kids would say, "What's wrong with Dad?" I would say something general, like "He's having a lot of emotional problems, but you'll have to talk to him about it." I didn't feel like I had the right to tell.

Keith and I had this ongoing fight about it. I'd say to him, "They're really worried about you. They're going to blame themselves." Finally, he decided to tell them. He sat down with the five older ones and told them everything, including the incident with his cousin. That really shocked me. I didn't think he'd tell them about the knife, but he did.

We apologized to the kids. We told them we were really sorry we had all this stuff from the past that was getting in the way of parenting them. They were really sweet. They said they thought we were great parents. It was a clearing out for all of us. He included them and I think it lifted something for them, too. They know it's not their job to take care of him, that this is something Dad has to deal with, with his therapist.

It has affected the kids. Our daughter, Judy, in particular. She was thirteen when Keith told her about the knife incident. Since then, every story she's written has had to do with death. She's quite an artist, and in our living room there's a rather surrealistic picture she drew of an alligator with a knife sticking out of it. It's gruesome, but it's her way of working it out.

We've only told Tommy, our youngest, a fraction of what we told the others. When he was six, and Keith wasn't working, I told him, "Daddy is sad and he's having some problems. He had a sad childhood." Keith and I have both said things like that to him, but we haven't told him any details. We don't want to scare him too much. He's still too young.

It's very much a part of Tommy's life that Daddy goes to his group, no matter what, and that Daddy and I are both in therapy. He asks me what I do there, and I say, "I sit and talk to Fran and then I feel better. You know how when you feel sad, and I ask you a question and you talk to me, you feel better?" He usually says, "Yes," and we can make a small parallel.

It's been confusing for Tommy. They had grandparents' day at school. All his friends have grandparents who give them dolls and toys and cars. My parents are dead. Keith's parents could care less. They've never wanted anything to do with the kids. Tommy told his teacher his grandparents were dead. I sat down with him and said, "Daddy's parents aren't really dead. They live far away. You've never seen them. They hurt Daddy, and they're not safe to be around. It's sad that you can't see them, but that's a decision Mommy and Daddy made. They aren't good people."

Sometimes I have trouble thinking I'm a good person because I picked somebody who has such a troubled history. I have felt deep guilt and remorse that I married and had children with somebody, not once, but twice, who struggles so much with his own demons that he can't give my children as much as they deserve. Keith is a good dad and the kids love him, but I've seen them suffer because of his moodiness and anxiety. Keith's had to keep quite a bit of distance at times, and that's hurt the kids. I've asked myself, "Why did I pick someone who couldn't give the optimal thing to me and to my kids?" I know the answer to that. It's what I was used to.

LEARNING TO BELIEVE IN CHANGE

My history has made me cynical. I've had to learn to believe in change. I never doubted that Keith would try very hard, but really believing he could change was hard for me. When I don't think there's hope for change, I start feeling frightened and boxed in. I see myself as an automaton repeating patterns. I started out with this pattern in my childhood and I can't seem to get out of it. I don't get my needs met. My children don't get their needs met. We're focusing on someone who's in crisis.

I don't know when the memories will ever end. The minute I struggle to accept one thing, there's more. It's like, "Okay, I got through physical abuse. I got through drowning. I got through sexual abuse. I got through murder. I got through multiple personalities." Now he has new memories. I'm scared it will never end, that this will be something he'll have to struggle with for the rest of his life, that he'll have to pull away from us for a few weeks while he's in a total panic, and we'll have to separate in order for me to survive emotionally and for him to get what he needs. Each time, it takes a toll, and I don't know what might be too much.

I keep thinking, "This is so horrible. Surely this is the last piece." When he remembered his cousin, he said, "This is the big piece. Everything fits now." It was horrible and we went through agonies, but there was the comfort that it was the last missing piece. And now there's more.

I want it to end. I want there to be no more new memories. I don't care about the old ones, but I want a promise that there aren't going to be any more, and of course, there's no promise. That's scary.

I can't say to Keith, "I'll be with you no matter what." It depends on how well I can handle it and how much he can give me at the time he's struggling through this, because I'm not in the mood to sacrifice my needs anymore. If he can't give me a decent amount, even though all my heart and sympathy are with him, we might have to separate. I think that in my scariest moments.

Most of the time now when he's in crisis, I don't focus on him. When he gets depressed now, he doesn't ask me to take care of him. He goes to other people. But I feel it. I love this man and I feel his pain in every pore of my skin. We're so close, I can feel it coming on. It affects me. I go through a difficult struggle to stay with my own positive feelings.

One thing that's helped is taking separate vacations. I was so enveloped in my first marriage that Keith and I made an agreement that I'd take time away every year. That has been a lifesaver for me. This spring was so hard. I spent a week in New Orleans with a woman friend. When I'm away, things fall into place for me. I get the perspective and solitude I need. If I didn't have the resources to get away, we wouldn't be together now.

The more I'm in crisis, the more I tend to think that things will fall apart and explode if I'm not around. The ability to say, "I'm going away. It's up to you," has been a real lifesaver. He has to take care of himself. He has to figure out how to feed the kids. And he's handled things beautifully every time. And we both feel more in love with each other when I return.

Spirituality has also helped me. I'm not a traditionally religious person, but when I started going to Al-Anon, I realized there was a hole in my life. I knew it wasn't going to be filled by going to church, so I've created my own spirituality. A lot of what I use is based on the 12-step model. Keith and I read a meditation to each other every morning. I also do a Native American ritual. We do some of everything. We have stuffed animals that we hug. I have every self-help book that was ever written. What helps me the most is spending lots of time in nature. I get connected to the earth. It renews me.

FORGING A COMMITMENT

For most of my life with Keith I said in the back of my mind, "You survived one marriage. If this doesn't work out, you can make it on your own." And I could. Financially, I'm independent. Yet this spring, when he was telling me all these terrible things that made me want to separate, it occurred to me that I really, really loved him and that it wouldn't be okay if we separated. I never let myself say that before. I used to say, "If he dies, I'd feel bad for awhile, but I'd make it." I used to think the only thing I might not survive would be the death of one of my children. But Keith and I have gone through so much together. He knows so much of me for so many years, and I know so much of him, that I really am invested. It's wonderful to know I've finally achieved some degree of intimacy, but terrifying because I never had that before in my life. I never trusted anyone enough to allow myself to feel this vulnerable. Aside from my children, this is a first. I'm committed to this relationship.

And that scares the shit out of me because if he can't change, if he has a breakdown, I don't know what I'll do.

But there has been change. He's proven it again and again. I've asked for something from him and I've gotten it. I've had to learn to ask for it. And most of the time Keith can give it to me, no matter what's going on.

Of course, I'd like him to keep getting better. I'd like him to get relief from the anxiety so he'll have the chance to fulfill more of his potential. But I think he's pretty terrific right now. I think I can live with him, as he is, forever. He's that much better. Things could get worse, I know, but if he could just be the way he is now for the rest of our lives, we'll do fine. Because I'm a realist. I don't expect perfection. I have good days and I have bad days. But mostly I get a lot from this man. Most of the time it's good between us and good with the kids. That's what really matters to me.

I've learned to believe in love. I've heard a lot of stories. I know there's a lot of horror and tragedy in the world. But I believe there's a way to connect to the good. I think people are capable of choice, capable of choosing the good. And the fact that Keith has never abused children, has never hit me, is so good a person, has never hurt anything in his life, when everything statistically says he should be a batterer or an abuser or a child molester, is a miracle. I see miracles like that all the time with people. People have faced almost insurmountable odds and chosen good. I believe in that.

I've learned that when this happens to you as a couple, it doesn't have to mean the end of your relationship. There's a way to work it through. When I choose to stay in this relationship and love Keith, I think I choose for other people, too. I'm showing that you can do more than just leave and run away. I'm showing that there's another choice. If I leave this relationship, it won't be because I'm afraid and I'm running away. It will be because it's the best thing for both of us.

HEALING BOOKS
AND OTHER
RESOURCES

Can you recommend any good reading material for partners of survivors that goes beyond saying, "Just be patient"?

FOR PARTNERS

(See also "Relationships" and "Sex")

Gil, Eliana. *Outgrowing the Pain Together: A Book for Partners and Spouses of Adults Abused as Children.* New York: Dell Bantam Doubleday, 1991.

Graber, Ken. *Ghosts in the Bedroom: A Guide for Partners of Incest Survivors.* Deerfield Beach, FL: Health Communications, 1991.
    A guide for partners that has a strong 12-step orientation.

Hansen, Paul. *Survivors and Partners: Healing the Relationships of Adult Survivors of Child Sexual Abuse.* Self-published.
    A positive, straightforward manual for couples. Send

Portions of this bibliography first appeared in *The Courage to Heal* and *The Courage to Heal Workbook.*

$11.00 (includes postage) to: Paul Hansen, 7548 Cresthill Drive, Longmont, CO 80501.

McEnvoy, Alan, and Jeff Brookings. *If She Is Raped: A Book for Husbands, Fathers, and Male Friends*. Holmes Beach, FL: Learning Publications (P.O. Box 1338, Holmes Beach, FL 34218), 1984.

Although written about adult rape, much of this book can be of value to partners of adults abused as children.

Maltz, Wendy. *Partners In Healing: Couples Overcoming the Sexual Repercussions of Incest*, 1988.

This excellent 43-minute video interviews several white, heterosexual couples about the effects of abuse on their sex lives. Includes practical suggestions for healing. Contact: Independent Video Services, 401 E. 10th Avenue, Suite 160, Eugene, OR 97401.

Mason, Patience H.C. *Recovering from the War: A Woman's Guide to Helping Your Vietnam Vet, Your Family, and Yourself*. New York: Penguin, 1990. This book focuses on the Vietnam experience, but offers valuable information on post-traumatic stress and being the partner of someone who's lived in a war zone, and survivors certainly qualify.

Strong, Maggie. *Mainstay: For the Well Spouse of the Chronically Ill*. New York: Penguin, 1989.

Written by a woman whose husband has multiple sclerosis, this powerful, practical, and beautifully written book raises many issues and feelings that will ring true for partners of survivors as well.

ABOUT SEXUAL ABUSE

Armstrong, Louise. *Home Front: Notes from the Family War Zone*. New York: McGraw-Hill, 1984.

Analysis of how we're doing in the war against child sexual abuse.

Bolton, Frank, Larry Morris and Ann MacEachron. *Males At Risk:*

The Other Side of Child Sexual Abuse. Newbury Park, CA: Sage Publications, 1989.

   A clinical book on the sexual abuse of boys.

Burns Maryviolet, M. Div, editor. *The Speaking Profits Us: Violence in the Lives of Women of Color/El Decirlo Nos Hace Bien A Nosotras: La Violencia en las Vidas de las Mujeres de Color.* Seattle: Center for the Prevention of Sexual and Domestic Violence (1914 N. 34th Street #105, Seattle, WA 98103), 1986.

   This much-needed collection of essays includes writing by Paula Gunn Allen, Tracy Lai, Evelyn White, Angela Ginorio, and Jane Reno, and talks about the relationships between violence and racism in the lives of Black, Latin, Asian and Native American women. Excellent. Written in Spanish and English.

Burson, Malcolm et al. *Discerning the Call to Social Ministry. An Alban Institute Case Study in Congregational Outreach.* Washington, DC: The Alban Institute (4125 Nebraska Avenue NW, Washington DC 20016), 1990.

   Case study that documents the exemplary handling of sexual abuse and domestic violence in one Maine church community. Also includes an excellent bibliography of materials relevant to churches grappling with family violence issues.

Butler, Sandra. *Conspiracy of Silence: The Trauma of Incest.* San Francisco: Volcano Press, 1985 (updated).

   A classic. Feminist analysis of child sexual abuse.

Crewsdon, John. *By Silence Betrayed: Sexual Abuse of Children in America.* New York: Little, Brown & Co., 1988.

Dziech, Billie Wright, and Judge Charles Shudson. *On Trial: America's Courts and Their Treatment of Sexually Abused Children.* New York: Beacon, 1989.

   An indictment of the justice system.

Family Violence Program, *Family Violence in Native Communities.*

   This bibliography lists references for books, articles, resources, and films that provide an overview of native culture and of family violence in native communities. To order, write: The Canadian Council on Social Development, 55 Parkdale Avenue, P.O. Box 3505, Station C, Ottawa, Ontario, CANADA K1Y 4G1.

Finkelhor, David. *Sexually Victimized Children*. New York: Free Press, 1979.

> Combines survivors' accounts with research data in a readable style. *Child Sexual Abuse: New Theory and Research* and *A Sourcebook on Child Sexual Abuse* are among the follow-ups.

Fortune, Marie. *Sexual Violence: The Unmentionable Sin: An Ethical and Pastoral Perspective*. New York: Pilgrim Press (475 Riverside Drive, Room 1140, New York, NY 10115), 1983.

> Written from a Christian and feminist point of view, this groundbreaking book looks at the reasons the church has ignored sexual abuse and rape, and explains why it is imperative for the church to change.

Hechler, David. *The Battle and the Backlash: The Child Sexual Abuse War*. Lexington, MA: Lexington Books, 1989.

> A well-researched journalistic investigation into the fight over child sexual abuse laws.

Herman, Judith. *Father-Daughter Incest*. Cambridge: Harvard University Press, 1981.

> A well-written, well-researched book about incest from a feminist perspective. This book does a good job of debunking long-standing myths.

Hunter, Mic. *Abused Boys: The Neglected Victims of Sexual Abuse*. Lexington, MA: Lexington Books, 1990.

> Solid. Well-researched. Hunter is also the editor of *The Sexually Abused Male Volume I & II*, an excellent two-volume collection of professional articles, published by Lexington Books in 1991.

Miller, Alice. *Thou Shalt Not Be Aware: Society's Betrayal of the Child*. New York: New American Library, 1986.

> A classic. Should be required reading for every therapist. Miller has written a number of excellent books, including *The Drama of the Gifted Child, For Your Own Good, Banished Knowledge*, and *The Untouched Key*.

Patton, Michael Quinn, editor. *Family Sexual Abuse: Frontline Research and Evaluation*. Newbury Park, CA: Sage Publications, 1991.

> Collection of clinical articles outlining current research on sexual abuse. Topics include: sibling abuse, female offenders,

sexual abuse in Native American families, and family reunification.

Pellauer, Mary, Barbara Chester and Jane Boyajian. *Sexual Assault and Abuse: A Handbook for Clergy and Religious Professionals.* San Francisco: Harper & Row, 1986.

    Varied essays give guidelines for a church response to sexual abuse.

Rossetti, Stephen. *Slayer of the Soul: Child Sexual Abuse and the Catholic Church.* Mystic, CT: Twenty-Third Publications (P.O. Box 180, Mystic, CT 06355), 1990.

    An anthology about the role of the church in dealing with child sexual abuse.

Rush, Florence. *The Best Kept Secret: Sexual Abuse of Children.* Englewood Cliffs, NJ: Prentice-Hall, 1980.

    An excellent feminist analysis of child sexual abuse from biblical times, to Freud, to the present.

Russell, Diana. *The Secret Trauma: Incest in the Lives of Girls and Women.* New York: Basic Books, 1986.

    The result of eight years of comprehensive incest research, this book shatters many previously held myths. Written in an academic style.

BATTERING

Fortune, Marie M. *Keeping the Faith: Questions and Answers for the Abused Woman.* San Francisco: Harper & Row, 1987.

    Primarily written for battered women, this clear, illuminating pamphlet is helpful for Christian women struggling to come to terms with God and with abuse in the home.

Gondolf, Edward, and David Russell. *Man to Man: A Guide for Men in Abusive Relationships.* Brandenton, FL: Human Services Institute (P.O. Box 14610, Brandenton, FL 34280), 1987.

    This simple, helpful volume is addressed to men who abuse

their partners. The book opens with a clear definition of wife abuse: "a husband's actions that destroy his wife's self-esteem," and goes on to explain how men can stop abuse. Written for men, this book can also help women abusers.

Island, David, and Patrick Letellier. *Men Who Beat the Men Who Love Them: Battered Gay Men and Domestic Violence*. New York: Haworth Press, 1991.

An important silence broken. Includes both theory and practical help.

Lobel, Kerry, ed. *Naming the Violence: Speaking Out About Lesbian Battering*. Seattle: Seal Press, 1986.

A landmark book that includes personal stories and explores the homophobia that has kept lesbian victims from reaching out for help.

Martin, Del. *Battered Wives*. Revised Edition. San Francisco: Volcano Press, 1981.

The pioneering book that framed the problem of wife-beating. Still the best overview available.

NiCarthy, Ginny. *Getting Free: A Handbook for Women in Abusive Relationships*. Seattle: Seal Press, 1986.

A practical, how-to guide for women wanting to leave an abusive partner. Valuable information on managing finances, housing, dealing with welfare, using professional help, evaluating feelings and needs. Expanded edition has sections on lesbian abuse, teen abuse, and emotional abuse. An easy-to-read edition, *You Can Be Free*, and an audio version are also available.

NiCarthy, Ginny. *The Ones Who Got Away: Women Who Left Abusive Partners*. Seattle: Seal Press, 1987.

A powerful chronicle of thirty-three battered women who got away from their abusive spouses.

Sonkin, Daniel Jay, Ph.D., and Michael Durphy, M.D. *Learning to Live Without Violence*. San Francisco: Volcano Press, 1989.

Designed as a handbook for men who batter women, this practical guide can help anyone who wants to deal with anger more effectively.

White, Evelyn C. *Chain Chain Change: For Black Women Dealing with Physical and Emotional Abuse.* Seattle: Seal Press, 1985.
> Direct and clearly written.

Zambrano, Myrna M. *Mejor Sola Que Mal Accompanada: Para la Mujer Golpeada/For the Latina in an Abusive Relationship.* Seattle: Seal Press, 1985.
> Bilingual. Excellent sections on institutionalized racism and barriers Latinas face in getting help.

RITUAL ABUSE

Believe the Children, P.O. Box 1358, Manhattan Beach, CA 90266.
> Provides resource materials, information, and a newsletter, as well as support for children who are victims of ritual abuse, and for their families.

Braun, Bennett, et al. *Ritual Child Abuse.* Cavalcade Productions, 1988.
> Thirty-minute video of clinicians discussing diagnosis and treatment for ritual abuse survivors. For information on rental or purchase of this or other videotapes on ritual abuse, write: Cavalcade Productions, 7360 Potter Valley Road, Ukiah, CA 95482. (800) 345-5530. In CA, call (707) 743-1168.

Families of Crimes of Silence, P.O. Box 2338, Canoga Park, CA 91306. (805) 298-8768.
> Provides resource information, support groups for *families* of abused children, trainings for professionals, and speakers on ritual abuse.

Hassan, Steven, *Combating Mind Control.* Inner Traditions, 1988. (Write: American International Distribution Corporation, 64 Depot Road, Colchester, VT 05466.)
> Talks about mind control used in cults and discusses ways to heal.

Healing Hearts, c/o Bay Area Women Against Rape, 1515 Webster Street, Oakland, CA 94612.

This organization offers an annotated bibliography, audio tapes of training conferences, and referrals for both professionals and ritual abuse survivors.

Kahaner, Larry. *Cults That Kill.* New York: Warner Books, 1988.
Written like a crime novel, this book explores cult crimes, primarily from a police viewpoint. Includes graphic stories by cult survivors.

Marshall Resource Center, Children's Institute International, 711 South New Hampshire, Los Angeles, CA 90005. (213) 251-4576.
Provides bibliography and articles on ritual abuse. Resource library open by appointment to survivors, partners, and professionals.

Morey, Terry. *The Ultimate Evil.* New York: Bantam, 1989.
Journalistic report on the "Son of Sam" trial in New York. Includes information on satanic rituals.

Ritual Abuse: Definitions, Glossary, the Use of Mind Control. Los Angeles County Commission for Women, 1989.
Write: L.A. County Commission for Women, 383 Hall of Administration, 500 W. Temple Street, Los Angeles, CA 90012. Available for $5.00.

Ritual Abuse Rap Line: (213) 534-4485.
This group also produces Raplines, a newsletter with a Christian emphasis.

Smith, Michelle, and Lawrence Pazder. *Michelle Remembers.* New York: Pocket Books, 1987.
First-person account of ritual abuse.

Spencer, Judith. *Suffer the Child.* New York: Pocket Books, 1989.
First-hand account of ritual abuse and resulting multiple personalities.

StarDancer, L. J. *Turtleboy and Jet the Wonderpup! A Therapeutic Comic for Ritual Abuse Survivors.* (To order, write to: StarDancer, P.O. Box 1284, Lakeport, CA 95453.) *Turtleboy* is $7.00, including postage. *Returning to Herself* is $9.00, including postage.
In graphic comic book style (that readers can color), a story of a child's heroic fight against ritual abuse. The graphic details

can evoke painful memories. Read with support, please. (Caryn StarDancer also has a book of poetry, *Returning to Herself*, about healing from ritual abuse.)

SurvivorShip: A Forum on Survival of Ritual Abuse, Torture & Mind Control. 3181 Mission Street #139, San Francisco, CA 94110.

SurvivorShip is a monthly forum on the survival of ritual abuse, torture, and mind control, reaching survivors and service providers across the U.S. and Canada. Includes articles by both professionals and survivors educating on all aspects of ritual abuse, including therapeutic strategies, book and conference reviews, interviews, prose, poetry, and art by adult and child survivors. Twelve monthly newsletters cost $30.00/year in the U.S.; $36.00/Canada. Back issues available for $3.00. A waiting list for subsidized survivor subscriptions is available.

MULTIPLE PERSONALITIES

Benson, Betty. *Shadow Lives*. New York: Bart, 1988.
Novel about a male survivor with multiple personalities.

Braun, Bennett. *Treatment of Multiple Personality Disorder*. Washington, DC: American Psychiatric Press (1400 K Street NW, Suite 1101, Washington, DC 20005), 1986.
Written for therapists, but still informative for the layperson.

Cohen, Barry, Esther Giller and Lynn W., editors. *Multiple Personality Disorder From the Inside Out*. Dallas: Sidran Press (Order Dept., 11271 Russwood Circle, Dallas, TX 75229), 1991.
Compiled by a therapist, a client, and a family member, this unique book addresses the complex issues of diagnosis, therapy, and maintaining personal relationships. Includes contributions and first person writings from over 150 people diagnosed with multiple personalities.

Gil, Eliana. *United We Stand: A Book for People with Multiple Personalities*. Walnut Creek, CA: Launch Press (P.O. Box 31493, Walnut Creek, CA 94598), 1990.
A wonderful, simple cartoon book that explains multiple

personalities and dissociation. A refreshing break from the usual sensationalism.

International Society for the Study of Multiple Personality and Dissociation.
Audiotapes of their meetings are available. Call Audio Transcripts, Ltd., at (703) 549-7334 for a catalog.

Investigations. Issues 3/4 of Volume 1, 1985. Edited by Brendan O'Regan.
A good overview of multiple personalities. Write: The Institute of Noetic Sciences, 475 Gate Five Road, Suite 300, Sausalito, CA 94965. ($4.50 + .75 postage; California residents add sales tax.)

Kluft, Richard. *Childhood Antecedents of Multiple Personality.* Washington, DC: American Psychiatric Press, 1985.
Clinical discussion of multiple personality development and treatment.

Many Voices: A National Bi-monthly Self-Help Publication for Persons with Multiple Personalities or a Dissociative Process.
Yearly subscriptions are $30.00. Write: Many Voices P.O. Box 2639, Cincinnati, OH 45201-2639. (Foreign subscriptions are $36.00.)

MPD Reaching Out: A Newsletter About Multiple Personality Disorder.
By MP patients currently in therapy. Subscriptions are $12.00. Write: c/o Public Relations Department, Royal Ottawa Hospital, 1145 Carling Avenue, Ottawa, Ontario, CANADA K1Z7K4.

Putnam, Frank. *Diagnosis and Treatment of Multiple Personality Disorder.* New York: Guilford Press, 1989.
Written for professionals, but useful for the lay reader, nonetheless.

Schreiber, Flora. *Sybil.* Chicago: Henry Regnery Co., 1973.
Classic story of extreme case of multiple personality.

The Troops for Truddi Chase. *When Rabbit Howls.* New York: E. P. Dutton, 1987.
Truddi Chase first developed multiple personalities when her stepfather raped her at age two. Written by her numerous

selves during therapy, this book intimately shows how the mind works to cope with the horror of sexual abuse. This book can be very hard to read.

ABUSE BY HELPING PROFESSIONALS

BASTA! Boston Associates to Stop Therapy Abuse. 528 Franklin Street, Cambridge, MA 02139.

> This organization offers workshops, support groups, consultation, advocacy, literature, training for professionals, support groups for partners, and other resources for people abused by helping professionals. Write for information.

Bates, Carolyn, and Annette Brodsky. *Sex in the Therapy Hour: A Case of Professional Incest.* New York: Guilford Press, 1989.

> A woman tells the story of abuse by her therapist.

Fortune, Marie. *Is Nothing Sacred? When Sex Invades the Pastoral Relationship.* San Francisco: Harper & Row, 1989.

> Case study of sexual abuse by a pastoral counselor.

Gabbard, Glen, ed. *Sexual Exploitation in Professional Relationships.* Washington, DC: American Psychiatric Press, 1989.

> An excellent collection of articles that deal with sexual misconduct by social workers, counselors, sex therapists, doctors, teachers, hospital staff, lawyers, and clergy. Guidelines for healing victims of abuse by professionals.

It's Never OK: A Handbook for Victims and Victim Advocates on Sexual Exploitation by Counselors and Therapists.

> This excellent booklet and its companion book for counselors can be ordered from: Minnesota Department of Corrections, Victim Services Unit, 300 Bigelow Building, 450 North Syndicate Street, St. Paul, MN 55104.

Pope, Kenneth, and Jacqueline Bouhoutsos. *Sexual Intimacy Between Therapists and Patients.* New York: Praeger, 1986.

> Comprehensive analysis of the problem. Suggestions for helping survivors of therapist abuse.

Rutter, Peter. *Sex in the Forbidden Zone*. New York: St. Martin's Press, 1989.

    A psychiatrist analyzes why so many men in power sexually exploit the women they're entrusted to help.

SURVIVORS SPEAK OUT

Anonymous. *Growing Through the Pain. The Incest Survivor's Companion*. Park Ridge, IL: Parkside Publishing, 1989.

    First-hand accounts by six women tracing their incest history and the beginning of their healing process.

Armstrong, Louise. *Kiss Daddy Goodnight: Ten Years Later*. New York: Pocket Books, 1987.

    An updated version of the classic speak-out on father-daughter incest. Armstrong challenges us to ask ourselves why incest is still going on and if we're doing enough to stop it.

Bass, Ellen, and Louise Thornton, eds. *I Never Told Anyone: Writings by Women Survivors of Child Sexual Abuse*. New York: Harper & Row, 1983.

    Vivid firsthand accounts of child sexual abuse.

Brady, Katherine. *Father's Days: A True Story of Incest*. New York: Dell, 1979.

    A first-person account of father-daughter incest.

Camille, Pamela. *Step On a Crack (You Break Your Father's Back)*. Chimney Rock, CO: Freedom Lights Press (P.O. Box 87, Chimney Rock, CO 81127), 1988.

Danica, Elly. *Don't. A Woman's Word*. Pittsburgh: Cleis Press (P.O. Box 8933, Pittsburgh, PA 15221), 1988.

    A powerful, gripping account from a survivor of sexual abuse and child pornography. A very hard book to read.

Donaforte, Laura. *I Remembered Myself: The Journal of a Survivor of Childhood Sexual Abuse*. Self-published. (For copies, send $7.00 to P.O. Box 914, Ukiah, CA 95482), 1982.

    Laura's journal details the struggles, pain, and triumphs of healing. This window into Laura's life offers a survivor's sense of humor and hope.

E. Nancy. *Once I Was a Child and There Was Much Pain: A Glimpse Into the Soul of an Incest Survivor.* San Francisco: Frog In The Well Press (P.O. Box 170052, San Francisco, CA 94117), 1988.
A powerful collection of drawings by a survivor.

Estrada, Hank. *Recovery for Male Victims of Child Abuse.* Santa Fe: Red Rabbit Press (P.O. Box 6545 Santa Fe, NM 87502-6545), 1990.
Clear, informative interview with a male survivor. ($7.00 includes tax and shipping; make checks payable to Hank Estrada.)

Evert, Kathy, and Inie Bijkerk. *When You're Ready: A Woman's Healing from Childhood Physical and Sexual Abuse by Her Mother.* Walnut Creek, CA: Launch Press, 1988.
A powerful resource for women molested by their mothers.

Grubman-Black, Stephen. *Broken Boys/Mending Men: Recovery from Child Sexual Abuse.* Blue Ridge Summit, PA: Tab Books (Human Services Institute, Inc., P.O. Box 14610, Brandenton, FL 34280), 1990.
Full of first hand accounts of men sexually abused as children, this healing book written by a male survivor is simple, clear, and helpful.

Incest. Speaking the Deadly Secret. People Productions Video, 2115 Pearl Street, Boulder, CO 80302. (303) 449-6086.
Despite the sensational title, this is a top-notch videotape. Sensitive and well-produced. Survivors use art and writing to talk about their pain and their healing. If you want to get inside a survivor's feelings, watch this tape.

McNaron, Toni, and Yarrow Morgan. *Voices in the Night: Women Speaking About Incest.* Pittsburgh: Cleis Press, 1982.
Women talk about their childhood experiences of abuse. Includes mother-daughter incest.

Morris, Michelle. *If I Should Die Before I Wake.* New York: Dell, 1982.
A harrowing fictional account of one woman's childhood experiences of incest. Guaranteed to evoke feelings and memories.

Randall, Margaret. *This is About Incest.* Ithaca: Firebrand Books (141 The Commons, Ithaca, NY 14850), 1987.

Using words and photography, Margaret Randall documents her healing from her grandfather's incestuous assaults.

Sessions, Shelly, with Peter Meyer. *Dark Obsession: A True Story of Incest and Justice.* New York: Putnam, 1990.

The true story of a successful suit against an incest perpetrator.

Thomas, T. *Men Surviving Incest: A Survivor Shares the Recovery Process.* Walnut Creek, CA: Launch Press, 1990.

A male survivor tells his story. Focuses on 12-step recovery.

White, Louise. *The Obsidian Mirror: An Adult Healing from Incest.* Seattle: Seal Press (3131 Western Avenue #410, Seattle, WA 98121), 1988.

A powerfully written description of the healing process from the inside out. Vividly describes the process of remembering and connecting with inner children. Graphic descriptions of abuse, however; you may need support.

ABOUT HEALING

Adams, Caren and Jennifer Fay. *Free of the Shadows: Recovering from Sexual Violence.* Oakland, CA: New Harbinger Publications, 1989.

Simple, clear, step-by-step guidance for rape victims. Excellent help for victims, families, and friends.

Barnes, Patty Derosier. *The Woman Inside: From Incest Victim to Survivor.* Racine, WI: Mother Courage Press, 1991.

This large format workbook is full of creative ideas and user-friendly healing strategies for women survivors.

Bass, Ellen, and Laura Davis. *The Courage to Heal: A Guide for Women Survivors of Child Abuse.* New York: Harper & Row, 1988.

A ground-breaker, this big book inspires, encourages, and informs. Written for women, but helpful to male survivors too.

Includes an in-depth section for partners. Also available on audio-cassette.

Bear, Euan, with Peter Dimock. *Adults Molested as Children: A Survivor's Manual for Women and Men.* Orwell, VT: Safer Society Press, 1988.

Excellent. A simple, straightforward approach to healing. The first to include women and men. (To order, send $12.95 to Safer Society Press, Shoreham Depot Road, RR1, Box 24-B, Orwell, VT 05760-9576.)

Blume, E. Sue. *Secret Survivors: Uncovering Incest and Its Aftereffects in Women.* New York: John Wiley & Sons, 1990.

A book that clearly delineates and describes the long-term effects of incest. Can help survivors discover that their experiences and reactions make sense.

Brady, Maureen. *Daybreak: Meditations for Women Survivors of Child Sexual Abuse.* San Francisco: Hazelden/Harper, 1991.

Affirming and inspiring.

Bronson, Catherine. *Growing Through the Pain: The Incest Survivor's Companion.* New York: Prentice Hall/Parkside, 1989.

Six women intimately describe their healing process.

Cole, Autumn and Becca Brin Manlove. *Brother-Sister Sexual Abuse: It Happens and It Hurts. A Book for Sister Survivors.* Ely, MN: Beccautumn Books (c/o Sexual Assault Program of Northern St. Louis County, 505 12th Avenue West, Virginia, MN 55792), 1991.

Based on Autumn Cole's doctoral dissertation, this clear and simple book validates the feelings, experiences, and healing needs of women who were molested by their brothers. Self-published. To order, send $7.95 for the book; $9.95 for an audio version. Add $2.00 for shipping.

Daugherty, Lynn B. *Why Me? Help for Victims of Child Sexual Abuse (Even if They Are Adults Now).* Racine, WI: Mother Courage Press, 1984.

A good, simple beginning book for child, teen and adult survivors.

Davis, Laura. *The Courage to Heal Workbook.* New York: Harper & Row, 1990.

Diverse in-depth exercises for men and women abused as children. Follows stages of healing outlined in *The Courage to Heal.* Designed for both individuals and survivors' groups. Includes exercises for sexual healing.

Davis, Nancy. *Therapeutic Stories to Heal Abused Children.* Self-published (Nancy Davis, 6178 Oxon Hill Road, Suite 306, Oxon Hill, MD 20745).

Originally written for therapists, this wonderful looseleaf book is full of healing bedtime stories and pictures to color. The big book is expensive; maybe you could share one. Some stories available on cassette too.

Engel, Beverly. *The Right to Innocence: Healing the Trauma of Child Sexual Abuse.* Los Angeles: J.P. Tarcher, 1989.

A recovery guide for adult survivors.

Gannon, J. Patrick. *Soul Survivors: A New Beginning for Adults Abused as Children.* New York: Prentice-Hall, 1989.

A clear, well-organized guide to healing for men and women. Deals with all types of abuse. Nice balance in emphasis between self-help and therapy. Includes a section for partners and one on parenting.

Gil, Eliana. *Outgrowing the Pain: A Book for and About Adults Abused as Children.* San Francisco: Launch Press, 1983.

An overview of the healing process from all kinds of abuse. Simple, clear text and cartoon illustrations make this book a good beginning resource. *Treatment of Adult Survivors of Child Sexual Abuse* is a guide for therapists.

Hall, Liz and Siobhan Lloyd. *Surviving Child Sexual Abuse: A Handbook for Helping Women Challenge their Past.* Philadelphia: The Falmer Press (Taylor & Francis Inc., 242 Cherry Street, Philadelphia, PA 19106), 1989.

A British book on healing. Full of helpful and interesting therapeutic and self-help techniques. Includes guidelines for group work.

Ledray, Linda. *Recovering From Rape.* New York: Henry Holt and Company, 1986.

An excellent guide for survivors of sexual assault, their partners, and families. Chapters on dealing with doctors, police, the legal system, emotional recovery and how to prevent rape. Although the book focuses on the immediate aftermath of rape, it deals with long-term consequences and includes a chapter for survivors of childhood abuse.

Lew, Mike. *Victims No Longer: Men Recovering from Incest and Other Sexual Child Abuse.* New York: Harper & Row, 1990.

Solid, clear, warm information and encouragement for men healing from child sexual abuse. A comprehensive, user-friendly groundbreaker.

Los Angeles Commission on Assaults Against Women. *Surviving Sexual Assault.* Chicago: Congdon and Weed, 1991.

An essential guidebook for survivors of sexual assault.

McClure, Mary Beth. *Reclaiming the Heart: A Handbook of Help and Hope for Survivors of Incest.* New York: Warner Books, 1990.

An affirming healing guide that draws strongly on 12-step traditions. Particularly valuable for survivors who are chemically dependent or from alcoholic homes.

Poston, Carol, and Karen Lison. *Reclaiming Our Lives: Hope for Adult Survivors of Incest.* New York: Bantam, 1989.

Nicely written, supportive healing guide by a survivor and therapist.

Ratner, Ellen. *The Other Side of the Family: A Book for Recovery from Abuse, Incest, and Neglect.* Deerfield Beach, FL: Health Communications, 1990.

A helpful workbook with a bias toward forgiveness and overcoming anger.

Sanders, Timothy. *Healing the Wounded Child: A 12-Step Recovery Program for Adult Male Survivors of Child Sexual Abuse.* Freedom, CA: Crossing Press, 1991.

Sanford, Linda. *Strong at the Broken Places: Overcoming the Trauma of Childhood Abuse.* New York: Random House, 1990.

Studies positive transformation in the lives of twenty survivors. Clearly focuses on the positive lives survivors can create out of the devastation of their childhoods. Empowering and empathetic.

Smith, Shauna. *Making Peace with Your Adult Children.* New York: Plenum, 1991.

> A practical, down-to-earth guide for parents struggling for better relationships with their adult children. Finally, a recovery book that encourages cross-generational healing.

W. Nancy. *On the Path: Affirmations for Adults Recovering from Childhood Sexual Abuse.* San Francisco: HarperCollins, 1991.

> Nancy W's affirmations are gentle, kind, and empowering.

Healing Organizations and Newsletters

Electronic Conference for Adult Survivors of Childhood Abuse, c/o Button and Dietz, Inc., P.O. Box 19243, Austin, TX 78760.

> Yes, a computer bulletin board for survivors and partners! Moderated by a therapist, this self-help resource is available twenty-four hours a day if you have a modem and a PC. Write for details. Beam up.

First Class Male, 50 N. Arlington Avenue, Indianapolis, IN 46219.

> Quarterly newsletter for sexually abused boys and men and the people who support them. Church-sponsored.

For Crying Out Loud, The Survivor's Newsletter Collective, c/o Women's Center, 46 Pleasant St., Cambridge, MA 02139.

> This fine quarterly newsletter is by and for women with a sexual abuse history. A one-year subscription costs $10.00.

Healing Paths, P.O. Box 599-SO, Coos Bay, OR 97420-0114.

> Eighteen dollars for a one year subscription. Bi-monthly.

Incest Recovery Association, 6200 North Central Expressway, Suite 209, Dallas, TX 75206. (214) 373-6607.

> Mental health professionals involved in treatment and education. Also provides a newsletter and some simple pamphlets. Groups for partners.

Incest Resources, 46 Pleasant Street, Cambridge, MA 02139. (617) 492-1818.

Provides extensive resources, legal information, professional education, and referrals.

Incest Survivors Information Exchange, P.O. Box 3399, New Haven, CT 06515.

This newsletter provides a forum for creative writing and creative sharing by survivors. Write for more information or for subscription rates.

Looking Up, P.O. Box K, Augusta, ME 04332. (207) 626-3402.

Looking Up is a national support organization for incest survivors. Provides referrals, resources, excellent publications, regional gatherings, and an outdoor adventure program.

Monarch Resources, P.O. Box 1293, Torrance, CA 90505, (213) 373-1958.

An informal clearinghouse which provides information (bibliographies, listings of newsletters, hotlines, support groups, referrals, and audio-visual resources) for each of four interest areas: childhood sexual abuse and incest, ritual abuse, multiple personalities, and partners and parents of survivors. Also publishes a quarterly calendar of events which lists upcoming conferences and workshops, and offers a speaker's bureau and a conference planning service. Nominal fee for written materials. Write or call for information. Long distance calls returned collect.

The National Child Abuse Help/IOF Foresters Hotline: 1-800-422-4453.

Provides twenty-four-hour crisis intervention and referrals. Call this number to report child abuse.

P.L.E.A., P.O. Box 6545, Santa Fe, NM 87502-6545. (505) 982-9184.

P.L.E.A. is the national organization for non-offending male survivors. Provides resources, a bibliography, referrals, and an excellent newsletter.

Serenity Quest: A Newsletter to Promote Growth and Healing, P.O. Box 2332, West Covina, CA 91723.

Newsletter for people in 12-step programs, many of whom are also survivors. Monthly. Subscriptions are $18.00/year. Free for people who can't afford the cost.

The Safer Society Program, Shoreham Depot Road, RR1, Box 24-B, Orwell, VT 05760. (802) 897-7541.

> National referrals and excellent literature available for both youthful and adult victim and offender populations. Send for a publications list.

SURVIVOR: A Creative Journal Created By Men and Women Survivors of Sexual Assault, Redbaux Communications, 3636 Taliluna, Suite 125, Knoxville, TN 37919.

> This super-glossy slick magazine welcomes writing and art submissions. Subscriptions are $12.00 for four issues.

The Survivor Network Newsletter, Box 80058, Albuquerque, NM 87198.

> A quarterly publication by, for, and about survivors. Subscriptions are $20.00/individual; $40.00/business professional; $10.00/underemployed. "Please contribute articles, poetry and artwork."

The Survivor Survivor Newsletter, P.L.E.A., P.O. Box 6545, Santa Fe, NM 87502-6545.

> This excellent quarterly newsletter provides a communication network and referral service for male survivors of physical, sexual, emotional abuse and neglect. Subscription cost is $20.00 for those who can afford it; less for those who can't.

Survivors of Incest Anonymous, P.O. Box 21817, Baltimore, MD 21222-6817.

> Provides free, confidential support meetings for survivors across the country. SIA and other 12-step programs have helped millions. To locate programs in your area, check the phone book, call a local social service agency, or request a directory of meetings from the national SIA number. Send a self-addressed stamped envelope with two stamps.

VOICES in Action, P.O. Box 148309, Chicago, IL 60614. (312) 327-1500.

> International organization for survivors and partners (called "pro-survivors"). Annual conferences, trainings, a newsletter, and an excellent program of special interest groups for networking around specific interest areas.

Women's Recovery Network, P.O. Box 141554, Columbus, OH 43214.

Puts out an excellent bimonthly newsletter for women survivors.

HEALING MUSIC

Nancy Day. *Survivor.* Available on cassette. Send $11.50 (includes postage) to Nancy Day, P.O. Box 8371, Pittsburgh, PA 15218.

Ruth Huber and Kate McLennan. *Trailblazers.* Available on cassette. Send $9.95 (includes postage) to Trailblazers, 7209 Grover Avenue, Austin, TX 78757.

Cathy Munsey-Kano. *NO MORE! Songs of Healing.* available on cassette. Send $10.00 (includes postage) to Heart Wings, 3128 Burr St., Fairfield, CT 06430, (203) 256-1094.

Fred Small. *I Will Stand Fast.* Title song is the theme song for partners everywhere. Available on record, cassette and CD. (Ask for Flying Fish #491.) Small's new album, *Jaguar,* (Flying Fish #570), features a powerful evocative song about incest, "Light in the Hall." Available on CD or cassette. To order, write to Roundup Records, P.O. Box 154, North Cambridge, MA 02140, or call 1-800-44-DISCS.

FOR PARENTS

ACT for Kids, Rape Crisis Network, 7 S. Howard, Suite 200, Spokane, WA 99204, (509) 747-8224 (PST).

ACT for Kids has produced many fine books, videos and other educational materials for children, parents, teachers, therapists, social workers, and other professionals who work with abused children. Of particular note is *My Very Own Book About Me* (available in Spanish and English), *How to Survive the Sexual Abuse of Your Child,* and *Giant Steps,* a self-esteem curriculum for children. ACT for Kids also produces fine training books and films for educators and for others whose job is to interview abused children. Call or write for a catalogue.

Adams, Caren and Jennifer Fay. *No More Secrets: Protecting Your Child From Sexual Assault.* San Luis Obispo: Impact Publishers, 1981.
A fine practical guide.

Bateman, Py, and Gayle Stringer. *Where Do I Start? A Parents' Guide for Talking to Teens about Acquaintance Rape.* Dubuque, IA: Kendall-Hunt Publishing, 1984.
Teaching teens about personal safety. Excellent sections on teens abused as children, and for parents who were victimized themselves.

Bettner, Betty Lou, and Amy Lew. *Raising Kids Who Can.* Newton Centre, MA: Connexions Press (10 Langley Road, Suite 200, Newton Centre, MA 02159), 1989.
A wonderful guide to empowering family meetings.

Byerly, Carolyn. *The Mother's Book: How to Survive the Incest of Your Child.* Dubuque, IA: Kendall-Hunt Publishing, 1985.
An excellent resource for women whose children have been molested.

Colao, Flora, and Tamar Hosansky. *Your Children Should Know.* New York: Harper & Row, 1987.
A top resource book for parents. Why, how, and when to talk to your children. What to do if assault occurs. Teaching children to be powerful.

Finkelhor, David, Linda Meyer Williams and Nanci Burns. *Nursery Crimes: Sexual Abuse in Day Care.* Newbury Park, CA: Sage Publications, 1988.
Research study of sexual abuse in day care centers. Discusses the extent of the problem, its wide-ranging impact, and makes suggestions for change.

Garbarino, James, Patrick Brookhouser, and Karen Authier. *Special Children—Special Risks. The Maltreatment of Children with Disabilities.* New York: Aldine de Gruyter (Aldine de Gruyter, Inc., 200 Saw Mill River Road, Hawthorne, NY 10532), 1987.
A clinical collection of essays on a critical topic.

Ginott, Haim. *Between Parent and Child.* New York: Avon Books, 1969.
> A classic.

Golder, Christine. *If It Happens to Your Child It Happens to You! A Parent's Help-Source for Sexual Assault.* Saratoga, CA: R & E Publishers (P.O. Box 2008, Saratoga, CA 95070), 1987.
> This large pamphlet deals effectively with many crucial parental concerns.

Gordon, Thomas, *P.E.T.: Parent Effectiveness Training.* New York: Peter Wyden Inc., 1970.
> This book has helped millions. Ground rules for good parenting.

Hagan, Kathleen, and Joyce Case. *When Your Child Has Been Molested.* Lexington, MA: Lexington Books, 1988.
> Simple, clear, and helpful.

Planned Parenthood. *How to Talk with Your Child about Sexuality: A Parent's Guide.* New York: Doubleday, 1986.
> Clear, direct and helpful. Includes a chapter on protecting your child from abuse.

Porter, Eugene. *Treating the Young Male Victim of Sexual Assault: Issues and Intervention Strategies.* Orwell, VT: Safer Society Press (The York State Council of Churches, Shoreham Depot Road, RR1, Box 24-B, Orwell, VT 05760-9756), 1986.
> A good basic book on the identification and treatment of young male victims of sexual assault.

Sanford, Linda. *The Silent Children: A Parent's Guide to the Prevention of Child Sexual Abuse.* New York: McGraw-Hill, 1980.
> Detailed and practical. Resources for single parents, parents of children with disabilities, parents who are Asian, Native American, Black, or Hispanic.

Schulenberg, Joy. *Gay Parenting: A Complete Guide for Gay Men and Lesbians with Children.* Garden City: Anchor Press, 1985.
> Practical and thorough. Readable. Includes a thorough resource section and bibliography.

COUNSELING AND SUPPORT GROUPS

Ernst, Sheila and Lucy Goodwin. *In Our Own Hands: A Woman's Book of Self-Help Therapy.* Los Angeles: J.P. Tarcher, 1981.

    Guidelines for starting a self-help group. Explores the politics of therapy and gives clear guidelines for picking a therapist. Feminist analysis of encounter groups, bodywork, massage, dance, psychodrama, gestalt, regression, and dream work. Practical exercises for each.

Gangi, Barbara, Fredda Bruckner-Gordon, and Gerry Wallman. *Making Therapy Work.* New York: Harper & Row, 1988.

    A guide to choosing, using, and ending therapy. Will help you evaluate and get the most out of therapy.

Hall, Marny. *The Lavender Couch: A Consumer's Guide to Psychotherapy for Lesbians and Gay Men.* Boston: Alyson Publications (40 Plimpton Street, Boston, MA 02118), 1985.

    The basics. Clear and simple with no therapeutic jargon or hocus-pocus.

Initiative, The Canadian Council on Social Development, 55 Parkdale Avenue, P.O. Box 3505, Station C, Ottawa, Ontario, CANADA K1Y 4G1.

    This excellent Canadian newsletter serves the self-help/mutual-aid community with current information and resources pertaining to self-help groups. Bilingual in English and French. Free in Canada. Write for information on U.S. subscriptions.

National Self-Help Clearinghouse, Graduate School, City University of NY, 33 West 42nd Street, Room 1222, New York, NY 10036. (212) 840-1259.

    Provides listings of self-help groups throughout the United States.

NiCarthy, Ginny, Karen Merriam, and Sandra Coffman. *Talking It Out: A Guide to Groups for Abused Women.* Seattle: Seal Press, 1984.

    Written with battered women in mind, this book offers a lot of sound advice about starting a group.

Webster, Linda, editor and compiler. *Sexual Assault and Child Sexual Abuse: A National Directory of Victim/Survivor Services and Preven-*

tion Programs. Phoenix: Oryx Press (2214 North Central at Encanto, Phoenix, AZ 85004-1483), 1989.

> An annotated guide to over 2,700 facilities. Designed for referral use. $55.00 Call 1-800-457-ORYX.

Westerlund, Elaine. *Starting from Scratch: The Incest Resources Group Model.* (Write: Incest Resources, 46 Pleasant Street, Cambridge, MA 02139.)

> A guidebook for starting self-help groups. Written for survivors; could be easily adapted for partners.

LEGAL RESOURCES FOR ADULT SURVIVORS

Kelvin and Patti Barton, P.O. Box 7651, Everett, WA 98201.

> This couple began researching the possibility of filing a civil suit against Patti's father in 1987. They were involved in the groundbreaking legislative changes which now enable adult survivors in Washington State to sue their perpetrators under the delayed discovery law.
>
> In the course of their research, the Bartons have become knowledgeable about the progress of delayed discovery legislation in all fifty states and are pushing for changes. They are eager to network with those working as advocates to change the laws nationwide. For information, send a self-addressed stamped envelope to the address above.

COVAC, 2111 Wilson Blvd., Suite 300, Arlington, VA 22201. (703) 276-2880.

> This is the coalition of victims' attorneys and consultants. They have extensive referrals and a database of all appellate cases involving victims nationwide.

The Incest Resources Legal Packet is full of information about cases involving child and adult survivors. Available for $12.95, includingpostage and handling. Write: Incest Resources, 46 Pleasant St., Cambridge, MA 02139. (617) 492-1818.

Greg Meyers, c/o Wise and Cole, 151 Meeting Street, Suite 200, P.O. Drawer O, Charleston, S.C. 29402. (803) 577-7032.

This lawyer has written guidelines that will help adult survivors who are thinking of suing their perpetrators.

National Center for Prosecution of Child Abuse, American Prosecutors Research Institute, 1033 North Fairfax Street, Suite 200, Alexandria, VA 22314.

Publishes monthly newsletter, UPDATE, which highlights the latest legal developments in regard to child abuse.

NOW Legal Defense and Education Fund, Intake Department, 99 Hudson Street, New York, NY 10013.

A clearinghouse of information on the legal rights of adult survivors of incest and child sexual abuse. Provides an excellent packet of information on legal issues and options. They do not handle cases themselves, but they do accept *written* requests for referrals of lawyers who handle sexual abuse cases in your area. No phone calls please.

RELATIONSHIPS

Beattie, Melody. *Codependent No More*. New York: Hazeldon, 1987.
This simple book launched a national movement.

Berry, Carmen Renee. *When Helping You Is Hurting Me: Escaping the Messiah Trap*. New York: Harper & Row, 1988.
Simple. Straightforward. Helpful. A refreshing lack of jargon.

Covington, Stephanie, and Liana Beckett. *Leaving the Enchanted Forest: The Path from Relationship Addiction to Intimacy*. New York: Harper & Row, 1988.

Hendrix, Harville. *Getting the Love You Want. A Guide for Couples*. New York: Harper & Row, 1990.
Harville's premise is that we all choose partners with whom we can work through our childhood pain. This excellent guide helps couples create a conscious partnership in which both partners can heal from old hurts.

Kritsberg, Wayne. *Healing Together*. Deerfield Beach, FL: Health

Communications, 1990.
>A healing guide for couples in recovery.

Lerner, Harriet. *The Dance of Anger*. New York: Harper & Row, 1986.
>Innovative ideas on how to deal with anger and communication in relationships. *The Dance of Intimacy* is the follow-up.

Mellody, Pia. *Facing Codependence*. New York: Harper & Row, 1988.

Schaef, Anne Wilson. *Escape from Intimacy*. New York: Harper & Row, 1989.

SEX

Bell, Ruth. *Changing Bodies, Changing Lives: A Book for Teens about Sex and Relationships*. New York: Random House, 1980.
>Although written with teens in mind, this nonsexist, nononsense guide can provide clear information for adult survivors learning about their bodies and healthy sexuality.

Blank, Joani. *The Playbook for Women About Sex*. Burlingame: Down There Press, 1982.
>A non-threatening, fun place to start a loving relationship with yourself. There is also a playbook for men.

Carnes, Patrick. *Out of the Shadows*. Minneapolis: CompCare Publishers, 1989.
>Landmark work that first identified and defined sexual addiction. Contrary to Love outlines treatment methods. Useful to professionals and recovering addicts. Based on a 12-step model.

Kasl, Charlotte Davis. *Women, Sex, and Addiction: A Search for Love and Power*. New York: Harper & Row, 1989.
>A powerful, ground-breaking book on women and sex addiction. Well-documented, well-thought-out, politically astute, and substantial. Kasl speaks with clarity, depth, and compassion.

Loulan, JoAnn. *Lesbian Sex*. San Francisco: Spinsters/Aunt Lute (P.O. Box 410687, San Francisco, CA 94141), 1984.
>Written for lesbians, but valuable for all women. Includes

information on sexual abuse. The follow-up, *Lesbian Passion,* has a chapter for partners.

Maltz, Wendy, and Beverly Holman. *Incest and Sexuality: A Guide to Understanding and Healing.* Lexington, MA: Lexington Books, 1987.

> An excellent resource for working through sexual (and other) problems individually and in a relationship. Includes guidelines for therapists and a brief section on male survivors.

Maltz, Wendy. *The Sexual Healing Journey.* New York: HarperCollins, 1991.

> A long-awaited book, this step-by-step sexual healing guide helps couples in which one partner is a survivor of sexual abuse. Top notch.

Mura, David. *A Male Grief: Notes on Pornography and Addiction.* Minneapolis, MN: Milkweed Editions (P.O. Box 3226, Minneapolis, MN 55403), 1987.

> A moving poetic essay that explores why so many men are addicted to pornography. Powerful, provocative, beautifully written.

Underwood, Judy, and Pamela Gaynor. *The Isle of Pleasure: Tapes to Guide Women to Sexual Fulfillment.*

> A self-paced series of six audio tapes for women survivors. There are two versions: heterosexual and lesbian. Six tapes cost $89.95 plus shipping. Maybe the members of a survivors' group could chip in for a set. Write: Odyssey, 515 S. Sherwood Street, Fort Collins, CO 80521.

Wells, Carol. *Right Brain Sex: Using Creative Visualization to Enhance Sexual Pleasure.* New York: Prentice-Hall, 1989.

> This interesting book helps you visualize yourself into a better sex life.

Mail-Order Stores for Vibrators, Sex Toys, and Other Books on Sex

Eve's Garden, Suite 420, 119 West 57th Street, New York, NY 10019.

> Send $2.00 for a catalog.

Good Vibrations, 1210 Valencia Street, San Francisco, CA 94110. Good Vibrations has two excellent mail-order catalogs: one for their top-notch Sexuality Library and one for sex toys. Send $2.00 for one, $3.00 for both.

MEN'S ISSUES

Abbott, Franklin. *New Men, New Minds: Breaking Male Tradition. How Today's Men Are Changing the Traditional Rules of Masculinity.* Freedom, CA: Crossing Press, 1987.

> Excellent, honest look at men, sex, and intimacy. The sequel, *Men and Intimacy: Personal Accounts Exploring the Dilemmas of Modern Male Sexuality,* is equally thought-provoking.

Bly, Robert. *Iron John: A Book about Men.* New York: Addison-Wesley, 1990.

> Alternative visions of men and masculinity which embrace the spiritual, emotional, and mystical aspects of life.

Keen, Sam. *Fire in the Belly: On Being A Man.* New York: Bantam, 1991.

> A thought-provoking exploration of manhood.

Lee, John. *Flying Boy.* Florida: Health Communications, 1989.

> A psychologist writes about the wounded child in men.

Pedersen, Loren. *Dark Hearts: The Unconscious Forces That Shape Men's Lives.* Boston: Shambhala Publications, 1991.

> A book that outlines the sources of men's pain and gives hope for healing.

The Sounds True Catalog: Special Men's Audiotape Supplement, 1825 Pearl Street, Boulder, CO 80302.

> Audiotape catalogue full of tapes from the leaders in the men's movement: Robert Bly, Robert Moore, Michael Meade, James Hillman, and more. For a copy of the catalogue, call toll-free, 1-800-333-9185.

Thompson, Keith. *To Be a Man.* Los Angeles: J.P. Tarcher, 1991.

> Essays on men and manhood.

NEWSLETTERS AND PERIODICALS

Changing Men, 306 N. Brooks Street, Madison, WI 53715.

> A magazine covering gender, sex, and political issues. Feminist viewpoint. Biannual. Subscriptions are $16.00/two years. Back issues $4.50.

Journeymen, 513 Chester Turnpike, Cania, NH 03034.

> A creative newsletter that talks about men's issues, spirituality, and sexuality. Quarterly. $24.00/year.

Man! 1611 W. Sixth Street, Austin, TX 78703.

> A journal from the Austin Men's Center. Focuses on relationships and recovery issues. Quarterly. $10.00/year.

Men Talk, 3255 Hennepin Ave South, Suite 45, Minneapolis, MN 55408.

> A newsletter from the Twin Cities Men's Center. Quarterly. $14.00/year.

Men's Council Journal, Box 4795, Boulder, CO 80306.

> A newsletter from the Colorado Men's Council. Includes art and poetry. Quarterly. $10.00/year.

Wingspan: A Journal of the Male Spirit, Box 1491, Manchester-by-the-Sea, MA 01944.

> A national publication devoted to exploring the male spirit. Large format quarterly. Write for details.

OTHER BOOKS OF INTEREST

Adams, Kathleen. *Journal to the Self: Twenty-two Paths to Personal Growth.* New York: Warner Books, 1990.

> A wonderfully clear and user-friendly guide to journalling. A gem for those of us who "get it out on paper" when we're searching to find our heart.

Black, Claudia. *It Will Never Happen to Me: Children of Alcoholics.* Denver: MAC Publishing, 1981.

> The first and still the best book for adult children of alco-

holics. Black has also published an excellent workbook for adult children, *Repeat After Me*.

Black, Claudia. *Double Duty*. New York: Ballantine Books, 1990.

> *Double Duty* examines the struggles of adult children from homes where chemical dependency and another factor—such as physical disability, sexual abuse, being gay or lesbian, being an only child, or eating disorders—make recovery more difficult.

Capaccione, Lucia. *The Picture of Health: Healing Your Life with Art*. Santa Monica, CA: Hay House (P.O. Box 2212, Santa Monica, CA 90406), 1990.

> A beautiful handbook and guide to art therapy.

Clarke, Jean Illsley and Carol Gesme. *Affirmation Ovals: 139 Ways to Give and Get Affirmations*. Plymouth, MN: Daisy Press (16535 9th Avenue, N. Plymouth, MN 55447), 1988. (Send $6.95 plus $2.50 postage to Daisy Press for ovals and accompanying handbook.)

> These affirmation ovals are wonderful reminders of the positive messages children should receive at each stage of their development. Great reminders for parents and for adults striving to build a more positive sense of self-esteem. Every survivor should have a set to play with. They're great! Daisy Press also offers an excellent variety of tapes, training materials, and other resources for building self-esteem. Write for more information.

Colgrove, Melba, Harold Bloomfield, and Peter McWilliams. *How to Survive the Loss of a Love*. New York: Bantam, 1976.

> A classic for dealing with grief and losses of all kinds. A day at a time, this simple, little book helps.

Davis, Martha, Matthew McKay, and Elizabeth Tobbins Eshelman. *The Relaxation and Stress Reduction Workbook*. Oakland, CA: New Harbinger Publications, 1982.

> A practical guidebook about nutrition, relaxation, meditation, self-hypnosis, assertiveness training, biofeedback, time management, and much more.

Dorris, Michael. *The Broken Cord*. New York: Harper & Row, 1989.

> A powerful, haunting memoir about a father's struggles with his son's fetal alcohol syndrome.

Groening, Matt. *Childhood is Hell*. New York: Pantheon Books, 1983.
Terrific cartoons about what childhood is really like.

Hagan, Kay. *Internal Affairs: A Journalkeeping Workbook for Self-Intimacy*. New York: HarperCollins, 1990.
A beautifully designed path to self-knowledge. Well-thought-out and deeply spirited. *Prayers to the Moon* is the beautiful follow-up volume.

Hendricks, Gay, and Russel Wills. *The Centering Book: Awareness Activities for Children, Parents, and Teachers*. New York: Prentice-Hall, 1975.
Designed for use with children, this simple book introduces you to the world of dreams, meditation, centering, body awareness, yoga, and guided imagery.

Hutchinson, Marcia Germaine, Ed.D. *Transforming Body Image*. Freedom, CA: Crossing Press, 1985.
Written for women. Step-by-step exercises help you integrate body, mind, and self-image.

Roth, Geneen. *When Food is Love: The Relationship Between Eating and Intimacy*. New York: Dutton, 1991.
A provocative, honest look at the relationship between compulsive eating, childhood pain, and intimacy. Roth's first book, *Feeding the Hungry Heart: The Experience of Compulsive Eating*, is an anthology about compulsive eating that looks at binging, hunger, and nourishment as issues far deeper than food. Her second, *Breaking Free*, offers practical guidelines to stop eating compulsively. Roth has also published a self-help workbook, *Why Weight?*

Sanford, Linda Tschirhart, and Mary Ellen Donovan. *Women & Self-Esteem: Understanding and Improving the Way We Think and Feel About Ourselves*. New York: Penguin Books, 1986.
Brilliant analysis of why women think poorly of themselves. Chock full of anecdotes and personal examples. "Blueprints for Change" at the end of each chapter offer useful exercises for anyone wanting to improve self-esteem.

Sher, Barbara, with Annie Gottlieb. *Wishcraft*. New York: Ballantine, 1979.

This book "makes hope practical." A guide for getting what you want in life, this book is a blend of "you-control-your-own-reality" ideology with practical goal-setting.

Silverstein, Schel. *The Missing Piece Meets the Big O*. New York: Harper & Row, 1981.

A classic storybook parable about relationships.

SOME CHOICE FICTION (FOR INSPIRATION)

Angelou, Maya. *I Know Why the Caged Bird Sings*. New York: Bantam, 1980.

A moving portrayal of incest and its effects, in a wonderful novel that celebrates life.

Barnes, Liz. *hand me downs*. San Francisco: Spinsters/Aunt Lute, 1985.

A delightful autobiographical novel written from the point of view of a spunky five-year-old who is abused by her brother.

Dickson, Margaret. *Maddy's Song*. Boston: Houghton Mifflin, 1985.

A beautifully written novel about a young girl's struggle to break free from a physically abusive father. Horrible, inspiring, and incredibly suspenseful, it's a tough book to put down.

Kingsolver, Barbara. *The Bean Trees*. New York: Harper & Row, 1988.

A wonderful novel about finding yourself, healing an abused child, and the power of love in a new "found" family. Kingsolver's second novel, *Animal Dreams*, is also a world of wonder.

LeGuin, Ursula. *A Wizard of Earthsea*. New York: Bantam, 1975.

Compelling fantasy story about a young man's quest to seek out and conquer the shadows that chase him. Survivors of sexual abuse will have no trouble identifying with his denial, his search, and his recovery.

Morrison, Toni. *The Bluest Eye*. New York: Pocket Books, 1970.

A beautiful novel about a young survivor.

Murphy, Patricia. *Searching for Spring*. Tallahassee, FL: Naiad Press (P.O. Box 10543, Tallahassee, FL 32302), 1987.

> This excellent novel explores the healing of one member of an incest group.

Swallow, Jean. *Leave a Light On for Me*. San Francisco: Spinsters/Aunt Lute, 1986.

> An inspiring novel about a lesbian relationship between an incest survivor and a recovering alcoholic that actually works out in the end.

Walker, Alice. *The Color Purple*. New York: Pocket Books, 1982.

> A young woman's letters to God. Triumph through adversity. Exquisite.

Zahava, Irene. *Hear the Silence: Stories of Myth, Magic, and Renewal*. Freedom, CA: Crossing Press, 1986.

> Diverse cross-cultural stories of women and spirituality. The first story is a knock-out about sexual abuse and retribution.

NOTE: An excellent mail-order source for hard-to-find abuse-related books is Full Circle Books in Albuquerque, New Mexico. For an extensive annotated bibliography on abuse, addiction, recovery, or eating disorders, send a self-addressed stamped envelope and $1.00 (for each bibliography requested) to Full Circle Books, 2205 Silver SE, Albuquerque, NM 87106.

INDEX

Abusers
  abused as, 19, 23–24, 124, 232–34
  confrontation of, 34, 215–17, 218,
    250
  denial by, 218
  directing anger toward, 61, 212,
    259
  as family member. *See* Family of
    abused
  help for, 232–33
  mixed feeling about, 213
  partner perceived as, 68
  partner's feeling about, 212, 213,
    215
  prosecution of, 120, 230
  protecting children from, 224–27,
    233, 251
  protection of, by survivor, 212–13
  punishment for, 120, 230
  reasons they get away with it, 120–
    21
  responsibility accepted by, 218–19
  siding with, 52
  telling your children about, 228–
    29, 251–52, 299–300
Acquired Immune Deficiency
    Syndrome (AIDS), 290–91

Addiction, 110
  alcohol abuse, 18, 132, 246–47,
    252–53, 293
  drug abuse, 18, 132, 296
  memories triggered upon recovery
    from, 116
Affairs, 280–81
Affection, 271, 286
Aging as trigger of memories, 116
Agreements, keeping, 155–56
Al-Anon, 55, 293, 302
Alcohol abuse, 18, 132, 246–47, 252–
    53, 293
Alcoholics Anonymous, 247, 253
Alters. *See* Multiple personalities
Anesthesia, 116
Anger
  abusive, 99–100
  directed at abuser, 61, 212, 259
  expressing, 79
  in healing process, 34
  misdirected, 95
  of partner, 34, 37, 61, 79, 212, 259
  physical outlets for, 34, 79
  self-mutilation to express, 110
  of survivor, 34, 95, 99–100, 110
Armstrong, Louise, 120*n*.

90, 208–10, 248–49, 255, 262, 267, 276–77, 282, 302–3
Communication, 254, 256–57, 281, 295
 lack of, 160–61
 limits on listening, 157–59, 253
 negotiation. *See* Negotiation
 partner's confiding information about the survivor, 32, 162–64
 during separations, 287
 talking about the abuser. *See* Talking about the abuse
Compassion, 16
Complaining, 169
Compromise, 167, 169
Confiding survivor's experience to others, 32, 162–64
Conflict, 167–68, 239
Confronting the abuser, 34, 215–17, 218, 250, 269
Conspiracy of Silence, The (Butler), 120*n.*
Contract, no-suicide, 112
Control in relationships, 151–52, 257, 263–64
 sex as means of, 199, 289–90
Coping skills of survivors, 92
Counseling. *See* Therapy and therapists
Courage to Heal, The (Davis and Bass), 29*n.*, 125, 196*n.*, 274
Courage to Heal Workbook, 106, 112, 196, 217*n.*
Courts, 120
Crewsdon, John, 120*n.*, 220*n.*
Crisis, constant, 92–94
Criticism, 165, 166
Cults, 13–14, 132–35
 Satanic, 111, 132–34, 260, 261, 262, 298–99
Culture
 abuse's root in, 127
 exploitation of sex, 82, 189

Danger, seeking out, 18, 19
Davis, Laura (author), 29*n.*, 125, 157, 196*n.*, 224

change in sexual feelings, 178
coping abilities, 92
flashbacks, 188–89
healing process for, 89
nighttime fears, 108
separation from partner, 88–89
sexual orientation, 205
Demands, stating needs versus making, 78, 167
Denial
 by abuser, 218
 by partner, 51–53, 267
 of partner's need to get involved, 52
 by siding with survivor's family, 52
 by siding with the abuser, 52
Dentists, memories triggered by, 116
Depression, 19, 101
 contact with family as cause of, 23
Disagreement, 167–68
Discerning the Call to Social Ministry: An Alban Institute Case Study (Burson et al.), 125*n.*
Disgust, 22
Dissociation, 20, 132, 136, 248, 259
Distancing, 146–48
Divorce, 175
Doctor visits, memories triggered at, 116
Drug abuse, 18, 132, 296
Dziech, Billie Wright, 120*n.*, 230*n.*

Eating disorders, 18. *See also* Weight change
Education, 24
Electric shocks, 261
Emergencies
 being there for, 84
 finding help for others in, 85
 self-mutilation, 109–10
 suicide. *See* Suicide
Emergency stage, 29–30
Emotional abuse, forms of, 232
Eric's story, 265–73
 Eric's background, 265
 partner support group, 268–69

Long-term effects of abuse, 18–25
  on body awareness, 20
  on family of survivor, 22–23
  on feelings, 19–20
  on intimacy, 21
  overcoming, 25
  on parenting, 23–24
  on self-esteem, 18–19
  on sexuality, 21–22
  on work, 24–25
Lorraine's story, 274–77
  ending the relationship, 276–77
Loulan, JoAnn, 185
Love, 303
  as end result, 175
Lovemaking. *See* Sex
Luci, story of Lorraine and, 274–77
  ending the relationship, 276–77

Making Peace with Your Adult Child
    (Smith), 231*n*.
Maltz, Wendy, 204
Manipulation, 169
Marriage counseling, 59, 246, 279,
    281
Massage, 116
Masturbation, 194, 203, 256, 271
Maurice's story, 254–57
  communication, 254, 256–57
  control, 257
  decision to stay together, 255
  sexual problems, 254, 255–56
  surfacing of Jo's memories, 254
Mediation, 253, 302
Memory(ies), 30, 260–61
  body, 268
  flashbacks. *See* Flashbacks
  incomplete, of abuse, 118–19
  repressed, 115
  surfacing of, 115–17, 254–259,
    266, 295–96, 298–99, 301
  triggers. *See* Triggers
  visual, 118
Men
  negative feelings about, 127–31,
    201–2

women's beliefs about sex drive of,
    201, 202
Miller, Alice, 124*n*.
Minnesota Department of
    Corrections, Counselors and
    Therapists of the, 141
*Mother's Book: How to Survive the Incest
    of Your Child* (Byerly), 230*n*.
Moulds, Robin, 136*n*.
Mourning, 33
Moving on, 34–35
Multiple personalities, 102, 103, 132,
    136–38, 260, 297
  as form of dissociation, 136
Music Box, The, 228–29

National Child Abuse Hotline, 233
Needs
  balancing partners' needs, 58–60,
    66–67, 72–74, 253
  conflicting, 167
  of couple who are both survivors,
    58–60
  listing your, 75–77, 170–71
  meeting your, variety of persons
    for, 76–77
  of partner, 66–67, 72–79, 253,
    262, 301
  ranking, 84–85
  recognizing your, 75–77
  sexual. *See* Sex
  stating of, versus making demands,
    78, 167
  See also Negotiation
Neglect, 232
Negotiation, 58, 72, 167, 169–74, 290
  action plans, 173
  choosing bottom lines, 171
  discussing lists of needs, 171–73
  ground rules for, 172
  lists of needs, 75–77, 170–71
  personal goals, 173–74
  poor alternatives to, 169
  ranking needs, 84–85
New Age spiritual beliefs, 125
Nightmares, 19, 107, 108, 279

Partners of survivors *(cont.)*
 multiple personalities. *See* Multiple
  personalities
 needs of, 66–67, 72–79, 253, 262,
  301
 negotiation. *See* Negotiation
 nighttime fears of survivor, 106–8
 "normal" relationship, desire for,
  143–44
 positive feelings of, 80
 protector role, 68
 questions of, 13, 236
 regression of survivor, 102–5
 safety and chaos, 145
 self-evaluation, 61–62, 272–73
 self-mutilation by survivor, 109–10
 sex. *See* Sex
 stories of, 243–303
 suicide and. *See* Suicide
 support for, 37, 39–40, 51, 207,
  209–10, 268–69, 279
 support from, 28, 34
 as survivor of abuse. *See* Survivor-
  survivor relationships
 survivor's self-absorption and, 36–
  38
 survivor unready to deal with the
  abuse, 54–55
 therapist abuse, response to, 140,
  268
 time off for, 84–85
 trustworthiness, 153–54
 violent behavior, 97*n*.
 why me?, 46–47
Patience, 16
Pedophiles, 82–83
Perfection, striving for, 18
Physical abuse
 forms of, 232
 Scott's story, 284–92
Pornography, 127
Powerlessness, 198
Prayer, 253
Pregnancy as trigger, 116, 259
Privacy, 162–64
Protector role of partner, 68

Punishment for abusers, 120, 230,
 268

Questions of partners, 13–236

Rage. *See* Anger
Rape, 127
Rape crisis centers, 106
Reality check, 93–94
Regression, 102–5
 duration of, 104–5
 explanation of, 102–4
 partner dealing with, 102–5
 therapist's role, 104, 105
Rejection, 201, 247, 248, 252, 255–
 56, 280, 287
Relaxation exercises, 104, 108
Religion, 253
 forgiveness and, 125
Remembering. *See* Memories
Repression of feelings, 19, 49
Resolution phase, 34–35, 124
Resourcefulness, 16
Revenge, desire for, 215, 250, 270
Richard's story, 278–83
 affairs, 280–81
 couple counseling, 279, 281
 family background, 278
 future thoughts, 282
 partner support group, 279
 reasons it's been worth it, 282–83
 sexual relationship, 278, 279, 280–
  81
Rigid behavior, 149–50
Ritual abuse, 13–14, 132–35, 260,
 261, 262. *See also* Satanic cults
Role models, 101, 265
Rossetti, Stephen, 125*n*.
Rules
 feeling rules of relationship have
  changed, 44–45
 inconsistent, 155
Rush, Florence, 120*n*.

Sadism, 203
Sadomasochism, 203

![HarperCollins logo] HarperCollins*Publishers*

To receive Laura Davis' free newsletter; to learn more about her books, workshops, and lectures; or to join her online healing community, visit www.LauraDavis.net

Books by Laura Davis (and Ellen Bass):

I Thought We'd Never Speak Again: *The Road from Estrangement to Reconciliation*
ISBN 0-06-019762-5 (HarperCollins hardcover by Laura Davis)

All of us carry the painful burden of relationships that have been sundered by betrayal, distrust, anger, and misunderstanding. In this groundbreaking new book, Laura Davis examines what tears people apart, what keeps them estranged, and lays out the steps by which they can mend broken relationships and find wholeness.

To find out whether reconciliation is possible or desirable for you, visit www.lauradavis.net/neverspeak2.asp

The Courage to Heal: *A Guide for Women Survivors of Child Sexual Abuse*
ISBN 0-06-095066-8 (paperback by Ellen Bass and Laura Davis) • ISBN 0-898-45833-1 (audio)

First published in 1988, this million-copy bestseller (now in its third edition) is an inspiring, comprehensive guide offering hope and encouragement to anyone who was sexually abused as a child. By taking readers step-by-step through the healing process with clarity, compassion, and a deep respect for each survivor's journey, *The Courage to Heal* can change your life and convince you that healing is possible—even for you.

The Courage to Heal Workbook:
For Women and Men Survivors of Child Sexual Abuse
ISBN 0-06-096437-5 (paperback by Laura Davis)

This groundbreaking companion to *The Courage to Heal* is an innovative, inspiring, and in-depth workbook containing checklists, open-ended questions, writing exercises, art projects, and activities that take survivors of child sexual abuse (or anyone suffering the effects of trauma) through the key aspects of the healing process.

Allies in Healing: *When the Person You Love Was Sexually Abused as a Child*
ISBN 0-06-096883-4 (paperback by Laura Davis)

Based on in-depth interviews, *Allies in Healing* speaks directly to the confusion, anger, bewilderment, and frustration of the partners of child sexual abuse survivors—girlfriends, boyfriends, spouses, and lovers—offering practical advice on deepening compassion, improving communication, and developing healing as a shared activity.

Beginning to Heal: *A First Book for Survivors of Child Sexual Abuse*
ISBN 0-06-096927-X (paperback by Ellen Bass and Laura Davis)

This gentle introduction to the healing process is perfect for teenagers, people in crisis, or anyone who wants to begin their journey of healing from sexual abuse.

Available wherever books are sold, or call 1-800-331-3761 to order.